Miscarriage
and The
Successful Pregnancy

Miscarriage and The Successful Pregnancy

✦

A Woman's Guide to Infertility and Reproductive Loss

William P. Hummel, M.D., F.A.C.O.G.

iUniverse, Inc.
New York Lincoln Shanghai

Miscarriage and The Successful Pregnancy
A Woman's Guide to Infertility and Reproductive Loss

iUniverse books may be ordered through booksellers or by contacting:

iUniverse
2021 Pine Lake Road, Suite 100
Lincoln, NE 68512
www.iuniverse.com
1-800-Authors (1-800-288-4677)

Note: this information is an attempt to provide guidance regarding the issues that may contribute to reproductive loss. This is not meant to replace representation by and consultation with medical professionals. Every effort has been made to ensure that the information contained in this book is complete and accurate. However, neither the publisher nor the author is engaged in rendering professional advice or services to the individual reader. The ideas, procedures and suggestions contained in this book are not intended as a substitute for a consultation with your physician. All matters regarding your health require medical supervision. Neither the author nor the publisher shall be liable or responsible for any loss or damage allegedly arising from any information or suggestion in this book.

ISBN-13: 978-0-595-35715-4 (pbk)
ISBN-13: 978-0-595-67262-2 (cloth)
ISBN-13: 978-0-595-80193-0 (ebk)
ISBN-10: 0-595-35715-6 (pbk)
ISBN-10: 0-595-67262-0 (cloth)
ISBN-10: 0-595-80193-5 (ebk)

Printed in the United States of America

To my loving wife Wendy and wonderful
children Mark, Scott and MacKenzie.
The miracles in my life!

Contents

Introduction

Growing up in a family of sisters, led me to find comfort and familiarity in the medical field of obstetrics and gynecology. As the exciting advances in reproductive technology developed with "test tube babies", I continued my medical training in reproductive endocrinology and infertility. Most patients refer to us as "infertility specialists" since we possess and provide the extra skills to achieve these "miracle babies" for deserving couples.

As a fertility specialist I see the depths of loss and joys of success everyday. It becomes clear that the goal of my life's work is a baby, not a pregnancy. Yet, as I looked for resources and support for my patients of reproductive loss, I was startled to find very little available. Most of my patients were too familiar with the well intentioned but trite words from friends: "it was meant to be". Even my medical colleagues would shrug their shoulders and say it must have been genetically abnormal or just "bad luck". Medicine itself finds it hard to refer to any particular specialist as "the" specialist for miscarriage. Patients on the other hand, continued to search for answers that weren't being offered.

It is in this context that I offer a book of support and medical insight into miscarriage factors that can be identified and corrected. The steps of evaluation uniquely empower women to bring forth to their doctors questions in search of an answer. Not that a single solution offers the desired result. Most of my experiences have lended support to a systematic and thorough evaluation. Most of my couples have several issues that add up…some are correctable and others not. But a thorough optimization of risk factors often brought success. Answers that offer renewed hope of dramatically increasing the chance of having a full term pregnancy and baby!

William Hummel, M.D.
San Diego Fertility Center
May 2005

PART I
Miscarriage—The Loss

1

The Natural History of Miscarriage

One of the keys to treating recurrent miscarriage is initiating the search for an answer. Many women who conceive will miscarry at some point and yet more than half of the pregnant women can have a successful pregnancy—even after three miscarriages. Since successful pregnancy may sometimes occur, it would seem that treatment might be unnecessary in some cases. However, women with certain risk factors such as advanced maternal age or a history of infertility benefit from an early, informed evaluation to optimize successful pregnancies and prevent additional reproductive loss.

Early pregnancy loss is the most common complication of human pregnancy, occurring in at least 75% of all women trying to become pregnant. Most of these losses are unrecognized and occur before or during the expected menses. The remaining 15% to 30% are spontaneous miscarriages or ectopic pregnancies diagnosed after clinical recognition of pregnancy. Most young, healthy women do not need evaluation because of one or even two miscarriages. Approximately 85% of women with a single spontaneous miscarriage will deliver a viable live infant in the next pregnancy. The chance for a successful pregnancy is highest if the woman has a history of one or more live births, and is reduced in women older than 35 years.

After a second pregnancy loss, couples naturally want to know the risk of yet another loss and what they can do to ensure a successful pregnancy. The clinical approach may offer insight, treatment or reassurance regarding the possible cause of the pregnancy loss. Often, a physician can offer emotional support and counseling as to treatment options available to you.

DEFINITION

The World Health Organization has defined spontaneous miscarriage as expulsion of an embryo or fetus weighing less than 500 grams, corresponding to about 20 to 22 weeks' gestation. The definition of recurrent miscarriage varies. Classically, the cutoff has been three or more spontaneous miscarriages. However, even two spontaneous pregnancy losses constitute "recurrent" miscarriage and may deserve evaluation. In a patient with a history of two miscarriages, the subsequent risk of pregnancy loss rises to about 25%, whereas 3 miscarriages raise the risk of a fourth miscarriage to 33%.

CAUSES

Determining the cause of recurrent miscarriage can be problematic. Losses during the first trimester are often (but not always) due to fetal genetic defects. Consecutive miscarriages in the same patient are not always due to the same reason. The causes of recurrent miscarriage can include implantation factors, genetic factors, autoimmune factors, endocrine factors, infection, and anatomic uterine abnormalities, to name a few.

Epidemiology of Infertility and Early Pregnancy Loss

Historically, children have been valued not only for social and psychological reasons but also because they perform essential economic functions. In agricultural societies, children, particularly sons, are needed to labor on the land, provide security for their parents in old age, and inherit the family land. In some religions children are essential so that they can pray for their ancestors. Thus large families have been equated with wealth and good fortune. Both historically and among some primitive societies today, childlessness has been attributed to divine punishment or a supernatural curse. The onus of a barren marriage has been particularly severe for women. In many societies a childless woman has become a social outcast and even a victim of superstition.

Industrialization, urbanization and economic pressure have led to smaller families being the norm. Higher education is no longer the exclusive domain of men. Women have increasingly joined the labor force to maintain their living standard or pursue professional ambitions. As a result, many couples are delaying childbearing, and some are choosing to remain childless.

Although scientific concepts have replaced many of the old belief systems regarding the causes and consequences of infertility, some of the traditional notions still abound. On the one hand, infertility still tends to be regarded primarily as a gynecologic problem. On the other, the belief that procreation is a sign of virility or a reflection of an individual's worth is not uncommon. Because most people in both traditional and modern societies want children, the inability to produce a child or the desired number of children is a significant, emotionally distressing problem for couples all over the world.

DEFINITION OF TERMS

The generally accepted clinical definition of infertility is the inability to conceive within 1 year of unprotected intercourse. Distinctions are made, however, between primary and secondary infertility. Primary infertility refers to a couple that has never achieved a pregnancy, whereas secondary infertility is used to describe a couple that has achieved at least one conception but is experiencing difficulties in achieving a subsequent pregnancy. Sterility usually means a complete and permanent inability to procreate. Reproductive loss is defined as an inability to carry a conceptus to a live birth and includes both spontaneous miscarriage and stillbirth.

MAGNITUDE OF THE PROBLEM

By using the clinical definition of infertility given above, two national surveys estimated that 11 percent of U.S. married couples were infertile in 1965 and 10 percent in 1976. Earlier census data, however, suggest that childlessness in some countries may be as high as 30 percent. Infertility as measured by the percentage of married women who have not had a child or pregnancy for a certain number of years in the absence of contraception is reported to be 17%.

Pregnancy loss represents the most common form of adverse reproductive outcome. Approximately 15 to 40 percent of recognized pregnancies end in spontaneous miscarriage. Most pregnancy loss occurs, however, before a woman is aware that she is pregnant. It has been estimated that as many as 40 to 60 percent of fertilized ova may not survive. Cases of early, unrecognized pregnancy loss generally cannot be distinguished from failures to conceive.

TRENDS IN INFERTILITY AND PREGNANCY LOSS

Because of limited data, it is not known if trends in infertility or pregnancy loss have changed over time. In the United States two national surveys indicate that infertility has increased slightly among young married women but not among older women seen from 1965 to 1976. The marked rise in sexually transmitted diseases represents a plausible explanation for the increase in infertility among young women. A substantial increase in demand for infertility services in the United States has also been documented, but this is thought to reflect the aging of the "baby-boom" generation, the postponement of childbearing and higher age-specific infertility rates.

Trends in pregnancy loss, particularly early losses, are equally difficult to ascertain. A longitudinal study of cohorts of college women concluded that there had been no change in spontaneous miscarriage rates for women who entered the study during 1935 to 1944 and those who enrolled a generation later during 1961 to 1970.

Natural History of Spontaneous Miscarriage

Experience with human in vitro fertilization (IVF) has shown that 10% to 30% of normal oocytes (eggs) do not fertilize, and another 10% to 50% fertilize but do not cleave or implant. About 15% to 40% of clinically detected pregnancies result in spontaneous miscarriage prior to 20 weeks' gestation. Thus, a fertilized oocyte has *at best* a 60% chance of reaching 20 weeks' gestation.

The data on sequential pregnancy losses cites a 13% risk of spontaneous miscarriage, with a greater risk noted if the couple had experienced a previous pregnancy loss. Women with previous live births experience similar proportions of reproductive loss. This increase in recurrent pregnancy loss risk may simply reflect the intensity with which subsequent miscarriage is diagnosed. Because many miscarriages are very early and often interpreted as slightly late menses, women with previous pregnancy losses are more likely to undergo close scrutiny for miscarriage than women with no known previous losses. The most important note is that without any treatment at all, the overall odds of a subsequent live birth are at least 23 to 33%. This has obvious impact for any demonstrated condition that "causes" recurrent pregnancy loss: many couples are likely not to abort again even with no specific treatment.

SUMMARIZING QUESTIONS AND ANSWERS

What is a miscarriage?

Miscarriage, or spontaneous miscarriage, is the loss of a pregnancy before the fourth month. The main symptoms are:

• Uterine bleeding

• Cramping of the uterus

• Passage of blood clots or tissue from the vagina

How often does a miscarriage occur?

Miscarriage is far more common than most women realize. About 15 out of 100 pregnancies end in miscarriage. Most of those miscarriages occur in the first three months of pregnancy.

Why does a miscarriage occur?

Over half of all miscarriages happen because the baby is not normal. We do know that miscarriage is NOT something that the mother has caused to happen.

How will I feel when I go home?
Normal symptoms that follow a miscarriage include:

• Bleeding—The type of bleeding may vary. You may stop after a few days or you may bleed on and off for several weeks. The bleeding should become less in amount each day and change from bright red to pink with more mucous. It is normal to pass clots. Keep in mind that when you lie down blood collects in your vagina. When you stand up this may pass in a large gush.

• Cramping—Minor low abdominal cramping is normal after a suction procedure. This will be more likely if you have had children. You may take two aspirin or Ibuprophen every four hours.

• Nausea—Nausea and some vomiting may occur with a suction procedure. This is fairly common and should pass within a few minutes.

- Grief and anger—These feelings are very common after a miscarriage. Some women feel guilty and try to think of a reason that could explain the miscarriage. It is important for you to be aware that neither you nor your partner caused the miscarriage. You should also know that having one miscarriage does not mean that the next pregnancy will have the same result.

You may find it helpful to talk to a friend or family member about your feelings. This is a time when you and your partner need support and care from those close to you. Many people who have had a miscarriage find a support group helpful. Your nurse may know of a support group in your area that includes other couples who have had a pregnancy loss.

Symptoms that aren't normal after a miscarriage:

- Bleeding which is more than a normal period. Soaking one maxi pad in one hour would be too much bleeding.

- Fever above 100.4° F or 38° C

- Vaginal discharge which smells foul or looks infected

- Low abdominal pain or tenderness lasting more than 24 hours

If these symptoms occur call a doctor or nurse!

Taking care of yourself after a miscarriage.

- Take your temperature two times daily for one week, in the late afternoon and at bedtime.

- Avoid intercourse, douching or tampons for at least two weeks. This is to prevent infection.

- You may take a shower as you wish.

- Slowly resume normal activities. You may return to work the next day unless your doctor tells you not to.

- If your blood type is Rh negative you may be given a shot of Rhogam to prevent problems with Rh disease.

• Make a follow-up appointment with your doctor.

HELPFUL HINTS FOR SUPPORTIVE FRIENDS AND FAMILY

What NOT to say.........

You can always have another child. At the moment, for most grieving parents, the most important child in the world is the wanted one they just lost and who can't be replaced.

It's for the best—the baby would have had to live with major health problems.

Stop crying. Crying is a normal and healthy part of the catharsis of grief. Failure to shed tears is not a sign of strength, but of shock or denial.

I know what you are going through. Unless you have suffered a similar loss, they will tend to resent your presumption.

2

The Emotional Impact of Reproductive Loss

PSYCHOLOGICAL FACTORS IN RESPONSE TO MISCARRIAGE

Grief is a common response to miscarriage. Women may experience shock, denial, psychological symptoms, anger, anxiety, guilt, and depression. The extent of this grief depends not on the duration of the pregnancy, but on the depth of the maternal attachment to the fetus. For women who have experienced multiple pregnancy losses, the emotional distress caused by each miscarriage may be cumulative, with increasing depression, grief and general unhappiness, and a sense of loss of control over reproductive options. Supportive physician evaluation and counseling may be one of the most important forms of treatment for women with recurrent pregnancy loss.

Couples should be prepared for the possibility of a pregnancy loss even before pregnancy is achieved. If a miscarriage occurs, the couple should be informed as to potential reasons for the loss and the risk of future losses. Couples may find it beneficial to meet with other couples or women who have experienced a similar loss.

The phenomenon of recurrent pregnancy loss can have an important and prolonged psychological significance. Because the loss is cumulative, it may create an enduring experience of unresolved grief that is essentially unique to couples that experience repeated reproductive loss. Couples suffering recurrent pregnancy loss, especially when no known medical cause has been found, must confront the reality of their functional infertility; as a result, their grief is compounded by the emotional devastation associated with the inability to carry a pregnancy to term. The psychosocial implications of this problem are complex, and for many couples, this recurrent loss has a profound effect on the tone and quality of their relationship.

Reaction to a miscarriage is very variable and once again there's no 'right' way to feel—a range of reactions are possible and normal. In addition to the grief you may feel, your body will be undergoing some profound hormonal adjustments, which may make you feel very emotionally fragile.

Grief is a very normal reaction to the loss you have experienced and it may be as intense as that after any other loss. Many women describe a feeling of numbness and emptiness following a miscarriage. Some couples withdraw, feeling alone and isolated, others may wish to talk about their loss.

Men often feel they have to be strong for their partner and find their loss particularly difficult to talk about. Although it is difficult at first, it may help to try and tell family or close friends how you feel.

HELPFUL HINTS FOR SUPPORTIVE FRIENDS AND FAMILY

- Do let your genuine concern and caring show.

- Do be available…to listen or to help with whatever seems needed at the time.

- Do say you are sorry about what has happened and about their pain.

- Do allow them to express as much unhappiness as they are feeling and are willing to share.

- Do encourage them to be patient with themselves and not to expect too much of themselves, nor to impose any 'shoulds' on themselves.

- Do allow them to talk about their loss as much and as often as they want to.

- Do reassure them that they did everything they could and that it wasn't their fault.

- Don't let your own sense of helplessness keep you from reaching out.

- Don't avoid them because you are uncomfortable. Being avoided by friends may add pain to an already painful experience.

- Don't say that you know how they feel (unless you have experienced their loss yourself, and then you can be particularly supportive).

- Don't tell them what they should feel or do.

- Don't change the subject when they mention their loss.

- Don't avoid mentioning their loss out of fear of reminding them of their pain (they won't have forgotten).

- Don't try to find something positive about the loss (e.g. a moral lesson, closer family ties, etc).

- Don't point out that at least they have their other....

- Don't say that they can always have another.... (They wanted this one).

- Don't say that they should be grateful for....

- Don't make comments that in any way suggest that the loss was their fault (there will be enough feelings of doubt and guilt already).

Grief

With any loss, there is a process that consists of three basic steps. The Grief Process:

(1) ***Shock/Denial***—"Oh, no! Not me!" "Oh, those can't be blood spots. I've been taking extra good care of myself."

(2) ***Anger/Guilt/Depression***—"Why me? If only I'd..." "I want a baby so much. Everyone else doesn't even care and they have perfect pregnancies." "I've felt sadder this week than ever in my life."

(3) ***Acceptance***—"Yes, me. It's part of my life and I have to deal with it. Many people lose pregnancies and somehow pull themselves together. Maybe one of them can give me information about a counselor or group to help me."

Each step takes longer to go through than the previous one. There are many setbacks; some are anticipated and others are unexpected. Setbacks may involve baby showers, birth experience stories, new babies, Ob/Gyn office visits, nursing mothers, thoughtless comments, holidays, and family reunions. These can gnaw at you and wear you down, or you can accept them as unavoidable temporary annoyances. Working through the grief process is a part of your healing. It will not erase the loss. You will not forget nor will you be the same as you were before. You will eventually find a comfortable place to tuck the memory of your loss.

How Others Might React

Most people aren't comfortable discussing loss or death. People who care a great deal about you often will react to your loss in a way that frustrates and disappoints you. They may not think of your loss as a death. They may not seem sympathetic about your sadness. There aren't many get-well cards for pregnancy loss. When dealing with others, you will only waste energy if you expect them to give more than they are able to give.

Some people might react with silence or avoidance. They may not even have known that you were pregnant. They may feel that they are intruding or are not well enough informed to talk with you about your loss. They probably feel certain that they'll say the wrong thing, and unfortunately that often is true. It doesn't occur to them that sending a "thinking of you" note, an "I'm sorry" card, a hug or small gift is appropriate and much better than remaining silent about your loss.

You will hear all about people who have endured and survived worse things. You will also hear comments like "Hurry and get pregnant again so you'll forget," or "It's for the best." Some people will try to figure out what you did wrong so that they can blame something for your loss. Incidentally, a surprising number of people will share their own loss experience with you. Be patient with them.

Supportive friends find books you should read, and take you out for lunch or shopping. You probably will appreciate this attention. It is easier to have someone with you the first few times you go out in public or the first day you go back to work. You will need to find the right balance with these helpers. You will need enough time to be alone as well as time to be alone with your partner.

In the medical arena be a wise medical consumer. Ask questions, take notes, make a list of questions and concerns. Learn to be carefully assertive and honest about your needs without being aggressive. For instance, you may have to request a follow-up visit with your doctor for test results mentioned in this book.

You and your partner's coping styles will probably be different. It will seem like you're on a seesaw. The woman often wants to review and mull over the loss and the male partner is more action-oriented and wants to get on with life. That doesn't mean he is not grieving. Partners don't always work through problems at the same pace or with the same solution. Often the woman is the consolee and her partner is the consoler. Neither partner should be the sole provider of support for the other. Although you will probably lean on one another at this time, each of you will need to find additional sources of support. Remind yourselves that you love each other. Take time together to be happy, to be sad, to talk, to hug, and then hug some more.

If you have other children in the family, they may blame themselves for your loss. Listen to their concerns and explain the truth at their level. They will need reassurance and probably some extra security, so that they won't be frightened about their own mortality. Allow them to be sad and also to see you sad.

Historical Perspective

Grief and the bereavement associated with the loss of a loved one have appeared in the literature but it was not until the 1970s that researchers began to investigate the mourning response in women who had lost a newborn. Kennel's classic study reported that women do indeed suffer severe grief reactions when they have had a reproductive loss. It was previously assumed that gestational age was the most important variable in predicting the severity and duration of a patient's reaction to early pregnancy loss and perinatal death. Thus, it was assumed that miscarriage and early pregnancy loss were less significant and less traumatic than stillbirth, and stillbirth was thought to be less significant than neonatal death. However, recent findings suggest that the degree of attachment to the pregnancy may in fact be a much better predictor of the severity of grief reactions than gestational age at the time of the loss.

Much has been written about a pregnant woman's attachment to the fetus when she first hears the fetal heartbeat or sees her first obstetrical ultrasound. Some have suggested that the use of reproductive technologies such as ultrasound have increased the pregnant woman's attachment to the fetus because they permit earlier bonding with the fetus. Others have suggested that new treatment technologies such as in-vitro fertilization (IVF) can allow observation of one's embryos and foster that attachment, thus leading to very early expectations about potential pregnancies. This sort of early attachment to the pregnancy, with its associated unrealistic expectations, may intensify the emotional impact of pregnancy loss.

NORMAL AND PATHOLOGIC GRIEF

The normal grieving process has common characteristics that include somatic distress, feelings of guilt and negligence regarding oneself. In most instances, this process dissipates within a few months and women are usually able to achieve a resolution of their grief and return to normal function and mood. Delayed grief (a postponement of the mourning process) occurs in persons who showed little or no sign of normal grieving immediately following the experience of loss, but who later suffered the full range of symptoms of mourning.

Pathologic grief may be witnessed in the form of distorted grief, and may represent a complication of the normal mourning process. Distorted grief may be described as maladaptive behavior in response to a loss. For example, a woman develops an exaggerated hostility toward pregnant women.

Perinatal Loss

Grief reactions following early pregnancy loss and death in the perinatal period differ from ordinary grief in certain common respects. Reproductive and perinatal loss is typically sudden and unexpected, and there are no established cultural and social responses to such a loss. The experience of the couple that has suffered such a loss is that it is "socially unspeakable"—that is, it is to be concealed and no public comment or response is required or appropriate.

Other factors that are unique to reproductive and perinatal grief reactions include the absence of an object to mourn (this is particularly true in the early pregnancy losses) and the unexplained nature of the loss. This is typically associated with intense guilt on the part of the woman regarding whether she herself caused the loss through some carelessness or indiscretion (e.g., some women believe that having sexual intercourse may have caused the pregnancy loss). In addition, couples suffering a perinatal grief reaction often experience reluctance on the part of friends and relatives to discuss the loss (leaving the couple feeling much more vulnerable and isolated). Conversely, comments by peers and relatives may be dismissive (e.g., "It was all for the best") rather than empathic and supportive. Other factors common in this type of loss include the unknown, unexpected aspect of the loss, the perceived need for each partner to appear strong for the other, and fears that the partner is not experiencing the loss in the "right way." In addition to the preceding factors women experiencing pregnancy loss feel a sense of betrayal by their own body, suffer intense feelings of vulnerability and loss of control, experience anger that an event that was anticipated with joy proved to be traumatic, and experience a sense of having failed.

Early Pregnancy Loss

It has only been in the past few years that early pregnancy loss (less than 12 weeks gestation) has been considered a significant cause of maternal grief. Although this reaction may not have the intensity of grief following stillbirth or neonatal death, it can have an important emotional impact that may be quite intense and may lead to unresolved and sometimes pathologic grief.

Several factors are unique to early pregnancy loss. Although guilt and a sense of helplessness are common in perinatal loss, a woman suffering early loss often has the experience of losing the pregnancy before she has even told anyone she is pregnant. As a result, she may be too embarrassed to discuss the pregnancy following the loss. On the other hand, if she has told others about the pregnancy, it may be an uncomfortable source of public communication informing others that she is no longer pregnant. Some women harbor ambivalent feelings about the pregnancy and this ambivalence may complicate reactions to early pregnancy loss, causing emotional confusion and guilt.

Gestational Age

The severity of grief reactions is not always directly related to the duration of gestation. Although pregnancy loss and perinatal death always appear to cause a grief reaction and all mothers seem to mourn, it appears that the degree of attachment to the pregnancy is most closely correlated with the intensity of the reaction.

There is a perinatal grief scale to assess the degree of maternal grief following pregnancy loss. The findings suggest that the intensity of attachment to the fetus provides the best explanation why the late-loss group typically registered more grief than parents in the early-loss group. As the pregnancy progresses and the reality gets closer, the experience of feeling the baby's movement can stimulate an intensified attachment. The ability to confirm pregnancy at earlier gestational ages combined with newer technologies such as ultrasound adds an earlier validation of this fetal bond.

As pregnancy progresses, couples have more time to plan, make announcements, and decide on a name for the baby, thus accentuating the bond. After the death of an infant in the second or third trimester, more women have an opportunity to hold the baby, to know the baby's sex, and have linking objects (such as a photograph of the baby, or the baby's hospital identification bracelet) and arranged for burial and a memorial service.

Recurrent Pregnancy Loss

The consequences for couples experiencing chronic miscarriage are often psychologically demanding and concerns unique to women who suffer recurrent pregnancy loss involve psychological implications for the couple's relationship. Both the cumulative grief of the repetitive pregnancy losses and the increasing ambivalence associated with the news of pregnancy cause ongoing emotional problems for couples in this frustrating dilemma. It appears that some degree of unresolved grief and guilt is inevitable after each loss, and each successive loss adds to an onerous cumulative burden. Women who have endured recurrent pregnancy loss frequently complain that they experience a continual sense of impending loss. The uncertainty about each pregnancy makes them increasingly ambivalent about each successive pregnancy. As a protective mechanism, women may distance themselves from a new pregnancy, beginning the bereavement process and separation from the pregnancy before an actual loss occurs but in anticipation of another failure.

In addition to this sustained intense ambivalence, feelings of loss of control, chronic anxiety, sleeplessness, loss of self-esteem, distorted body image, and a loss of libido. Similarly, partners in this situation commonly report feelings of helplessness, lack of control, anger, guilt, and an acute loss of self-esteem. As the reproductive losses accumulate, men increasingly doubt the value and meaning of continuing attempts at having a child and its impact upon their relationship. The accumulated burden of this ambivalence and anxiety can lead to situational impotence and fear of sexual relations.

Infertility

Infertility and its treatment may represent an emotionally difficult time for couples, affecting their marital, sexual, familial, and social relationships. Infertility is defined as "the inability to conceive a pregnancy after a year of sexual relations without contraception." If women are over the age of 35, this definition is

reduced to "six months of sexual relations without contraception." This acknowl-
edges the impact of a woman's age and its genetic impact on the egg, when assessing this transition from reproductive loss to infertility.

Couples that suffer recurrent pregnancy loss and infertility experience unique
stresses. On one hand they achieve distanced envy by couples who cannot achieve
pregnancy, to only feel isolated in their expectation of impending loss when pregnant.

Women with infertility share the sense that there is something wrong with
them. This sense that they are reproductively defective often contributes to their
distorted self-image, body image, and sense of themselves as sexually whole and
desirable. The experiences of isolation, anger, and guilt are common to couples
who experience infertility or reproductive loss. They often feel that their situation
is "out of control" and that they are alone in a baby-oriented world.

Aside from these broad similarities, the psychological aspects of infertility and
recurrent pregnancy loss have important differences. Couples who are unable to
conceive cling to and are consoled by the continuing hope that they will conceive, and that once that goal is achieved, they will be able to have a child. They
can view conception without ambivalence as the immediate goal of their efforts.
Couples suffering recurrent pregnancy loss inevitably regard conception with
increasing ambivalence, and they are unable to approach the pregnancy without a
great deal of anxiety. As women of reproductive age delay their family, we see
more couples that share a conglomeration of the above two groups. Once able to
conceive and experience loss while now unable to conceive at all.

In summary, there is a growing population of couples in whom the woman is
over 35 years of age and has experienced multiple pregnancy losses complicated
by subsequent infertility. The psychosocial impact of recurrent pregnancy loss
and infertility leave couples with unresolved grief, depression and poor self-
esteem. These experiences represent significant stress upon a couple's relationship
and the realization of whether they will be able to have a family of their own.

Residual Grief and Past Pregnancy Losses

Women with a history of past pregnancy losses are more likely to suffer a severe
grief reaction following subsequent pregnancy losses. If a woman has a history of
having difficulty conceiving and then loses a pregnancy, the grief reaction may be
quite severe. Any woman who has lost a pregnancy is likely to experience ambivalence and anxiety when embarking on a new pregnancy. In most instances, however, the woman reaches a point when she begins to feel secure about the new

pregnancy and her anxiety and ambivalence begin to subside as she passes new obstetrical milestones.

CASE REPORT

WJK, a 35-year-old married woman with a history of three consecutive pregnancy losses within 2 years, requested treatment with an infertility specialist because, after the third loss she had not been able to conceive for 8 months. She stated "There must be something terribly wrong with me! I am afraid I'll never be able to have a baby."

After treatment with follicle stimulating hormone (FSH) and progesterone support, the fertility center was pleased to report to WJK that her pregnancy test was positive. However, the nurses became confused and baffled when WJK cried uncontrollably when she heard the news. When the fertility center referred her to the psychologist for counseling and support, WJK said that she was flooded with feelings of ambivalence and fears about the possibility of yet another loss. She insisted that she could only feel fear about the pregnancy and, although she tried, she could not "feel joy about it."

Chronic Depression

Residual unresolved grief may cause clinically significant depression. The woman who suffers one loss after another may be confused about her reactions and feelings. After a single pregnancy loss, women frequently can remember every detail of the event and of the pregnancy. However, women who suffer from recurrent pregnancy loss are often confused about the focus of their grief. This cumulative grief is particularly acute when grief over individual losses has been minimized or unacknowledged. For example, a woman who had lost four pregnancies in a little over a year with very little time to grieve between pregnancies said that she could remember with incredible clarity the minutest details of each pregnancy loss. However, she added that in her recollection, the pain, anger, and guilt she felt each time were blurred together and vague. Instead of mourning a series of specific losses, she felt continually unhappy and forlorn without a clear sense of how much was contributed by any one loss.

CASE REPORT

DL was referred to the psychologist after her husband reported that he was extremely worried about his wife's depression. After her third pregnancy loss, DL stopped going out of her house, gained weight, and was frequently tearful. Her husband said that he had grown accustomed to her constant distress but that he was exhausted by the effort involved in constantly trying to reassure her. DL said that she was beginning to feel that she had nothing to live for. She was unable to connect her emotional state directly to the pregnancy losses but rather felt that her life had been a series of disappointments and that there was little prospect that the future offered any likely improvement in her situation. However, she was able to acknowledge guilty ruminations concerning her possible role in the pregnancy losses. She said that she found that she was always angry with her family because they were constantly trying to cheer her up admit that it was "for the best".

The Couple

Women have been reported to grieve more than men in part because their attachment to the pregnancy is greater and because the mother is in fact grieving for a "part of herself." Attachment to the pregnancy often develops later for men than it does for women, so the spouse of a woman who suffers recurrent early pregnancy losses may have a much different emotional response and may therefore be at a loss to understand the intensity and duration of his wife's reactions. This is particularly true when the loss is early in the pregnancy; e.g., when the woman suffers a miscarriage, "some husbands feel less affected by the miscarriage than their wives because the pregnancy was not yet a physical reality for them.

As men and women experience pregnancy differently, they also grieve differently, which is not to suggest that there is no grieving on the part of the men. Men frequently complain about feeling lost in the process, of not knowing how to behave. They complain that they want to be the strong, supportive partner. However, at the same time, they are frequently confused and at a loss as to how to respond, and they may have only a limited understanding of the experience and treatment that their wives have undergone.

When to Stop Trying

The unresolved ambivalence that is a result of the repetitive pregnancy loss and/or infertility can result in confusion and uncertainty about future family planning. Fertility specialists have diagnostic tests that quantitate the chance of success for each unique couple. Some issues may not be "treatable" such as a woman's advanced age. Other diagnosis may be very treatable, such as a uterine septum, and result in a very optimistic prognosis. The emphasis is empowering the couple to seek the evaluation and care of a fertility specialist with whom they request a list of the factors that are likely to be responsible for their losses and a subsequent treatment plan and the prognosis with which it associates. An honest relationship with a physician should supply this insight and at times associate a percentage of likely success to be expected. Couples then reserve the right to discuss the implications of these insights and numbers, to make an informed decision to move forward with treatments or explore alternatives such as adoption, egg donation and gestational surrogacy.

INFORMATION ABOUT SUPPORT GROUPS

Couples can often derive considerable support and reassurance from those who have had similar experiences. National support groups such as Empty Cradle and Resolve have chapters in many local communities. These groups have reading material available that describes the grieving process to people who experience these losses so that they know that their behavior is normal. Information is also available for those couples who may be ready to discuss other alternatives, such as adoption, egg donation and gestational surrogacy.

Planning Your Next Pregnancy

After a loss, making the decision to try another pregnancy can be difficult. Seek a consultation with a medical specialist about the causes of your loss and how they might influence a future pregnancy. You might want to consult a geneticist, infertility specialist or perinatologist (a high risk obstetrician). Deciding when to attempt a pregnancy is a decision only the partners involved can make after a thorough medical evaluation has been completed. Treatments such as preimplantation genetic diagnosis (PGD) may have addressed genetic concerns, otherwise thought untreatable. It takes medical insight and a strong relationship for both partners to be ready to conceive again. It isn't easy but the rewards are there for those who endure with supportive medical care.

Your next pregnancy should probably be monitored with more attention. Your pregnancy may be viewed as one requiring "special" attention, but not necessarily a "high risk" pregnancy. Fertility treatments, hormone support and ultrasound monitoring may do wonders for a different obstetrical experience.

Individuals will make suggestions about what you should do to make your precious pregnancy successful. Some people do this because they also identify with your pregnancy and are emotionally invested in your pregnancy. The easiest way to handle their suggestions is to listen, and then follow your doctor's recommendations.

Your birth experience might be challenged by memories that resurface about your previous losses, especially if you are at the same hospital and with the same medical staff. You probably will need to do some grieving in addition to celebrating the new life.

Delayed bonding can be a natural outcome of your previous loss. You may feel the need to protect yourself from more sorrow so you might be cautious with your bonding until you're certain that all is safe and sure with your new baby. Don't worry if you don't bond immediately, it will come in time.

YOU CAN SURVIVE PREGNANCY LOSS

Most people have not learned coping skills for grief and loss. Pregnancy loss may be your first personal encounter with death. Surviving a loss is hard work; grief exhausts your endurance. Healing does happen in time. Focus on getting through the grieving rather than on the suffering.

Be receptive to the caring and support of others and be patient with their shortcomings. While you are learning a lot about death, you are also learning a lot about life. Your reading of this information means you are on a path that will lead you through the struggle to survival. You can survive your pregnancy loss.

"THE TRUTH IS…"

- **The truth ISN'T that you will feel "all better" in a couple of days, or weeks, or even months.**
  The truth IS that the days will be filled with an unending ache and the nights

will feel one million sad years long for a while. Healing is attained only after the slow necessary progression through the stages of grief and mourning.

- **The truth isn't that a new pregnancy will help you forget.**
  The truth is that while thoughts of a new pregnancy soon may provide hope, a lost infant deserves to be mourned just as you would have with anyone you loved. Grieving takes a lot of energy and can be both emotionally and physically draining. This could have an impact upon your health during another pregnancy.

- **The truth isn't that grieving is morbid or a sign of weakness.**
  The truth is that grieving is work that must be done. Allow yourself the time. Try not to fight it too often. It will get easier if you expect that it is variable, that some days are better than others. Be patient with yourself—there are no short cuts to healing. The active grieving will be over when all the work is done.

- **The truth isn't that grief is all consuming.**
  The truth is that in the midst of the most agonizing time of your life, there will be laughter. Don't feel guilty. Laugh if you want to. Just as you must allow yourself the time to grieve, you must also allow yourself the time to laugh. Viewing laughter as part of the healing process, just as overwhelming sadness is now, will make the pain more bearable.

- **The truth isn't that one person can bear this alone.**
  The truth is that while only you can make the choices necessary to return to the mainstream of life a healed person, others in your life are also grieving and are feeling very helpless. As unfair as it may seem, the burden of remaining in contact with family and friends often falls on you. They are afraid to "butt in," or they may be fearful of saying or doing the wrong thing. This makes them feel even more helpless. They need to be told honestly what they can do to help. They don't need to be told, "I'm doing fine" when you're really NOT doing fine. By allowing others to share in your pain and assist you with your needs, you will be comforted and they will feel less helpless.

- **The truth isn't that God must be punishing you for something.**
  The truth is that sometimes miscarriage just happens. This was not an act of any God; it was an act of Nature. It isn't fair to blame God, or yourself, or anyone else. Try to understand that it is human nature to look for a place to put the blame. Sometimes there are answers and sometimes there are not. Believing that you are being punished will only get in the way of your healing

- **The truth isn't that you will be unable to make any decisions during this time.**
It will be difficult, but decisions dealing with the death of your baby (seeing and naming the baby, arranging and/or attending a religious ritual, taking care of the nursery items you have acquired) are all choices you can make for yourself. Well-meaning people will try to shelter you from making these decisions; however, these first decisions are very important. They help to make the loss real. Our brains filter out much of the pain early on and soon after that, we find ourselves reliving the events over and over, trying to remember everything. This is another way that we acknowledge the loss. Until the loss is real, grieving cannot begin. Being involved at this early time will be a painful experience, but it will help you deal with your grief better as you progress by providing comforting memories of having performed loving, caring acts for your baby.

- **The truth isn't that you will be delighted to hear that a friend or other loved one has just given birth to a healthy baby.**
The truth is that you may find it very difficult to be around mothers with young babies. You may be hurt, or angry, or jealous. You may wonder why you couldn't have had that joy. You may be resentful, or refuse to see friends with new babies. You want someone to understand how it feels. You may also feel very ashamed that you could wish such things on people you love or care about, or think that you must be a dreadful person. You aren't. Forgive yourself. These feelings will eventually go away.

- **The truth isn't that all relationships survive this difficult time.**
The truth is that sometimes you might blame one another, resent one another, or dislike being with one another. If you find this happening, get help. There are self-help groups available or grief counselors who can help. Don't ignore it or tuck it away assuming it will get better. It won't. Talking it out with others may help. It might even save your marriage.

- **The truth isn't that eventually you will accept the loss of your baby and forget all about this awful time.**
The truth is that acceptance is a word reserved for the understanding you come to when you've successfully grieved the loss of a parent, or a grandparent, or a beloved older relative. When you lose a child, your whole future has been affected, not your past. No one can really accept that. But there is resolution in the form of healing and learning how to cope. You will survive. Many of us who have gone through this type of grief are afraid we might forget about our babies once we begin to heal. This won't happen. You will always remem-

ber your precious baby because successful grieving carves a place in your heart where he or she will live forever.

3

The Six Types of Miscarriage

BLIGHTED OVUM

A blighted ovum is a pregnancy in which cells develop to form the pregnancy sac, but not the embryo itself. An egg is fertilized and attaches itself to the uterine wall, but the embryo doesn't develop further. Blighted ovum pregnancies are the cause of about 50 percent of first-trimester miscarriages. There may be no bleeding to signal a problem and the hormones of pregnancy are frequently within a normal range.

A woman may not realize she has a blighted ovum until her doctor performs an ultrasound revealing an empty gestational sac. A blighted ovum can be the result of chromosomal problems. In some cases, the egg or the sperm may be of poor quality. In the past, many women miscarried a blighted ovum pregnancy without knowing what had happened. Today, technologies such as ultrasound can examine exactly what is going on inside the uterus so the diagnosis is becoming more common due to improved diagnosis. The management of a blighted ovum pregnancy is similar to that of a miscarriage (see below).

ECTOPIC PREGNANCY

A pregnancy in which the fertilized egg implants in tissue outside of the uterus and the placenta and fetus begin to develop there is called an ectopic pregnancy. The most common site of an ectopic pregnancy is within a Fallopian tube; however, ectopic pregnancies can occur in the ovary, the abdomen, and in the cervix.

Ectopic pregnancies are usually caused by conditions that obstruct or slow the passage of a fertilized ovum (egg) through the Fallopian tube to the uterus. This may be caused by a physical blockage in the tube, or by failure of the tubal epithelium to move the zygote down the tube and into the uterus. Most cases are a result of scarring caused by previous tubal infection. Up to 50% of women with ectopic pregnancies have a medical history of a tubal infection (salpingitis) or pelvic inflammatory disease (PID). Some ectopic pregnancies can be traced to congenital tubal abnormalities, endometriosis, pelvic scar tissue caused by a ruptured appendix, ruptured ovarian cysts and prior ectopic pregnancies.

On occasion, a woman will conceive after elective tubal sterilization. The risk of an ectopic pregnancy occurring in this situation may reach 60%. Women who have had surgery to reverse previous tubal sterilization in order to become pregnant also have an increased risk of ectopic pregnancy (when reversal is successful).

The incidence of ectopic pregnancies ranges from 1 in every 40 to 100 pregnancies. Increased risk is associated with women who have a history of salpingitis and/or PID, tubal surgery of any type (including tubal ligation and reversal of a tubal ligation), or prior ectopic pregnancy.

Tubal pregnancies, which make up the majority of ectopic pregnancies, may be prevented by avoiding those conditions that cause scarring of the Fallopian tubes. Such prevention may include avoiding risk factors for PID (multiple partners, intercourse without a condom, and contracting sexually transmitted diseases) and early diagnosis and adequate treatment of salpingitis and pelvic inflammatory disease (PID).

Symptoms of an ectopic tubal pregnancy may include:

- lower abdominal or pelvic pain

- mild cramping on one side of the pelvis

- amenorrhea (cessation of regular menstrual cycle)

- abnormal vaginal bleeding-usually scant amounts

- breast tenderness

- nausea

If rupture and hemorrhaging occurs before successfully treating the pregnancy, symptoms may worsen and include:

- Severe, sharp, and sudden pain in the lower abdominal area

- feeling faint or actually fainting

- referred pain to the shoulder area

Diagnosing an Ectopic Pregnancy

- Tenderness in the region of the tube or ovary on the affected side

- There is usually a positive pregnancy test

  - Urine HCG (qualitative) tests may be falsely negative in up to 17.5% of them.

  - In contrast, serum HCG (quantitative) tests have only a 2% incidence of false negative results.

- A hematocrit test may be normal or decreased

- The white blood cell count may be normal or increased

- An ultrasound illustrates an empty uterus. Products of conception may be evident elsewhere.

- A laparoscopy and or a laparotomy may be necessary for adequate diagnosis

Treatment

In the event that pelvic-organ rupture has occurred because of the ectopic pregnancy, internal bleeding and/or hemorrhage may lead to shock. Nearly 20% of ectopic pregnancies present themselves in this manner. This is an emergency condition.

Surgical laparotomy is performed to stop the internal bleeding (in cases in which rupture has already occurred), confirm the diagnosis, and remove the non-viable products of conception. In non-emergency cases, mini-laparotomy or laparoscopy may be alternative surgical methods. Such alternatives have similar outcomes; however, they are less invasive and are available at a lower cost because they require minimal hospitalization or outpatient treatment.

Non-surgical (medical) management is being implemented for very early ectopic pregnancies without suspected immediate danger of rupture. In such cases, methotrexate is a medication administered with careful outpatient monitoring of the woman and serial quantitative HCG and CBC levels followed.

Expectations after an ectopic pregnancy

About 50% of the women who have experienced an ectopic pregnancy are later able to achieve a normal pregnancy. A subsequent ectopic pregnancy may occur in 10 to 20 % of cases. Some women fail to become pregnant again, while others become pregnant and spontaneously abort during the first trimester.

SPONTANEOUS MISCARRIAGE IN THE 1ST TRIMESTER

Spontaneous miscarriage is the loss of a pregnancy before the fetus is 12 weeks gestational age. Spontaneous miscarriage in the first trimester occurs in about 30% of pregnancies and frequently occurs so early that the woman is unaware that she is pregnant. Most miscarriages occur during the first 12 weeks of pregnancy. Many miscarriages are only "threatened," and the pregnancy continues to term, although symptoms may be the same.

Some causes of reproductive loss during the first 3 months (first trimester) include:

• An abnormal fetus

• Uterine abnormalities that prevent the fertilized egg from growing normally

• Use of drugs that harm the fetus

• Infections, especially virus infections, such as rubella or influenza

Risk of spontaneous miscarriage increases with:

• Stress; poor nutrition

• Illness that has lowered resistance

• Recent serious infection

• Medical history of endocrine diseases, such as diabetes mellitus or hypothyroidism

Preventing a spontaneous miscarriage includes eating a well-balanced diet and the avoidance of alcohol, cigarettes or recreational drugs. Don't use any medications, including non-prescription drugs, without consulting a doctor.

Diagnostic measures:

- Medical history and exam by a doctor

- Ultrasound

A doctor's treatment may include the following:

- Surgery: D & C (dilatation and curettage) or D & E (dilatation and evacuation) to remove any remaining tissue or the dead fetus

- The administration of a medication to induce the spontaneous expulsion of uterine contents of non-viable products of conception

Possible complications:

- Uterine infection, signaled by fever, chills and aching; hemorrhaging from other body parts

- "Incomplete" abortion, in which some placenta or fetal tissue remains in the uterus, or missed abortion, in which the fetus dies but remains in the uterus

Final Thoughts

- An inevitable miscarriage cannot be stopped.

- With treatment, a miscarriage is not a life-threatening condition. It usually does not affect a woman's ability to carry a healthy baby to term in the future

- Feelings of loss and grief are common. If these persist, seek emotional help.

Medication:

- Your doctor may prescribe: Oxytocin to control bleeding in some patients.

- Pain medication if needed.

- After a miscarriage, antibiotics for infection

- Blood transfusions for severe blood loss

- RhoD (immune globulin) for Rh-negative female

Threatened Miscarriage

For a threatened miscarriage, follow your doctor's orders. Bed rest is often enough to stabilize the pregnancy. After a miscarriage: Expect a small amount of vaginal bleeding or spotting for 8 to 10 days. Don't use tampons for 2 to 4 weeks. Wait through several normal menstrual cycles (usually 2 to 3) before attempting to become pregnant. Your doctor will advise you.

Activity:

For a threatened miscarriage: Rest in bed until symptoms disappear. Avoid sexual intercourse until the outcome is known.

Call your doctor if any bleeding occurs during pregnancy.

- Bleeding and cramps worsen during a threatened miscarriage or you pass tissue

- Fever and chills occur during a threatened miscarriage or following miscarriage

- Unexplained bruising occurs after a miscarriage

- Infection develops while you are pregnant

MOLAR PREGNANCY

A molar pregnancy is a rare abnormal pregnancy that affects 1 in every 2000 pregnancies. There is an increased risk after age 40, but the incidence is still quite low. In a molar pregnancy, an abnormal mass forms inside the uterus instead of a live fetus. Molar pregnancies are caused by an abnormality in the chromosomes of the sperm that fertilized the egg or the egg itself.

A molar pregnancy puts a woman at risk for the development of a malignant tumor in the uterus. While the risk is low, the tumor is highly invasive and highly metastatic. Therefore, any woman who has had a molar pregnancy requires careful monitoring after the molar pregnancy is removed. In the event that a malignant tumor develops, early treatment with chemotherapy has a success rate of nearly 100%.

Signs and Symptoms of a Molar Pregnancy

• Vaginal bleeding in the early weeks of pregnancy (almost always by week 12)

• Uterus larger than normal size for date of pregnancy

Diagnosis of a Molar Pregnancy

Most molar pregnancies are diagnosed during the first trimester. The physician makes the diagnosis based on the presence of bleeding, ultrasound, and lab values. Blood levels of human chorionic gonadotropin (HCG), a normal hormone of pregnancy, are abnormally high in a molar pregnancy. An ultrasound exam by the doctor will visualize the uterus to see whether a normal fetus or a hydatidiform mole is developing.

Treatment of Molar Pregnancy

A molar pregnancy is removed. Most commonly, suction curettage is done. During this procedure, the cervix is dilated and the uterine contents are removed with gentle suction. A woman is sedated during the procedure.

Since a molar pregnancy carries a small risk of the development of a malignancy, follow up care is quite important. The doctor will monitor the HCG level for a period to ensure that it returns to zero. In the event of a malignancy, the HCG level remains high or even increases after the pregnancy is terminated. For this reason it is important not to conceive again until your doctor approves.

Future Pregnancies

A woman who has had a molar pregnancy will probably be advised to postpone pregnancy for at least a year. Molar pregnancy carries the risk of the development of a malignant tumor in the uterus. While the risk is rare, any woman who develops a tumor and requires chemotherapy should discuss fertility issues with her cancer specialist.

INCOMPETENT CERVIX

An incompetent cervix is suggested by a history of mid-trimester pregnancy loss without antecedent uterine contractions. Several diagnostic techniques have been suggested to assess the integrity of the nongravid cervical canal, such as examination with Hagar dilators or an inflated Foley catheter. The efficacy of these methods has not been established.

Fetal loss in the second trimester in the absence of antecedent labor requires a detailed history regarding prior pregnancy outcomes and possible DES exposure. A painless second-trimester miscarriage in the face of an otherwise normal evaluation suggests cervical incompetence. Instrumentation of the cervix, including conization and dilation and curettage, or a traumatic vaginal delivery, may predispose to cervical incompetence.

Exposure to DES in utero has been clearly associated with an increased risk of second-trimester pregnancy loss. The mechanism by which this occurs is primarily cervical incompetence, although a T-shaped uterine cavity may also increase the risk. The diagnosis of DES-related anatomic abnormalities is suggested by a hysterogram demonstrating a dilated cervical canal or a T-shaped uterine cavity.

Treatment of an incompetent cervix consists of cerclage placement and restriction of activity. Cerclage, whether accomplished by the Shirodkar or Macdonald technique, is highly effective. Because the Macdonald technique has less associated morbidity and is generally simpler to perform, it is preferred by most practitioners.

Prophylactic cerclage for DES-exposed patients has been advocated, even in the absence of prior pregnancy loss. This recommendation is based on a study of 61 women exposed to DES in which 25 had a prophylactic cerclage and 36 were observed. In the group who underwent prophylactic surgery, 88% of pregnancies resulted in term delivery. Sixteen of the 36 who did not have prophylactic surgery required emergency cerclage; the subsequent term delivery rate in this group was 75%. Of the remaining 20 patients who did not undergo surgery, 70% were delivered at term. These results suggest that prophylactic cerclage may be warranted in DES-exposed patients.

STILLBIRTH

What Is Stillbirth?

Stillbirth and miscarriage both define a pregnancy loss. Stillbirth is the death of a baby after the 20th week of pregnancy but prior to delivery. Most often it is detected while the baby is in the mother's uterus, sometimes not until labor is underway. Miscarriage (sometimes called spontaneous abortion) is a loss that occurs before the 20th week of pregnancy.

There is a great sense of disappointment and loss whenever parents suffer the death of their baby, whether it is an early pregnancy loss, a late pregnancy loss, or a loss occurring sometime after birth. Stillbirth and miscarriage are separately defined, not because one is an easier or more difficult loss with which to deal, but because they differ in many ways. Stillbirth and miscarriage have different causes, need different evaluations, and differ medically and in the ways that parents and families can best be helped.

Stillbirth is common. It may affect anyone. There is no way to predict when stillbirth will happen or who will experience it. Stillbirth occurs in families of all races, religions, and income levels. Each year in the United States about 25,000 babies, or 68 babies every day, are born still. This is about 1 stillbirth in every 115 births. Something as common as this will, at some point, directly or indirectly touch the lives of many people. A friend, a relative, or you, yourself, may experience stillbirth.

Why Do Stillbirths Happen?

One of the most common questions following a stillbirth is, "Why did my baby die?" Answering this question is not always easy or possible. Extensive and careful examination of the baby and placenta is needed following delivery. Often these evaluations will provide helpful information and eventually bring peace of mind. With extensive evaluation, a cause for stillbirth can be identified in 40%-50% of all stillbirths. Even when a cause is not specifically identified, at least potential high risks for recurrence may be ruled out. Parents who experience stillbirth will be asked to consider extensive evaluations for their baby. Many will want everything done to try to discover why their baby died. Others may think that such assessment violates their baby. The decision should be theirs. Couples will need to choose what is best for them.

Causes of Stillbirth

Information about cause can be very important for parents and families. It may help parents in planning future pregnancies by providing insight to the frequently asked question, "Will stillbirth happen again?" The information may also help parents and families to deal emotionally with their loss. Knowledge, in general, can be empowering, and it may provide a sense of comfort by helping to alleviate uncertainty or guilt.

Identifiable causes of stillbirth generally fall into one of three different categories: birth defects in the baby, problems with the placenta or umbilical cord, or maternal illnesses or conditions, which may sometimes affect pregnancy.

• Birth defects are common but often overlooked causes for stillbirth. About one-fourth of babies who are stillborn have one or more birth defects that are responsible for their death.

• The placenta and umbilical cord is the baby's "lifeline" for oxygen and nutrients. Problems in either one may completely cut off or severely interfere with the needed flow of blood, oxygen, and nutrients to the baby. Although commonly pointed to as the likely cause for the death of a baby, problems with the placenta or umbilical cord actually account for only a moderate number of stillbirths.

• Although uncommon, maternal conditions may be responsible for stillbirth. Certain illnesses in the mother, such as diabetes or hypertension, and their treatments, sometimes cause stillbirths. An increased risk for stillbirth is also associated with the use of certain recreational drugs, particularly cocaine.

In addition, there are many other rare causes of stillbirth. Stillbirths are usually not caused by something parents or family members did or did not do.

Some Common Responses to Stillbirth

In the natural course of life events, babies are least of all expected to die. The loss of a baby through stillbirth can be overwhelming and devastating for parents as well as for family members and friends. Although such feelings are surprising to some, the stillbirth of a baby is a great loss, as great as that of an older child or any loved one.

When stillbirth occurs, parents who were anxiously awaiting a baby suddenly are not. It is natural for them to grieve deeply for the baby who has died and for the hopes, dreams, and wishes that will never be; hopes, dreams, and wishes that, for parents, are real long before the birth of their baby. They may feel a strong sense of sadness, or anger, or bitterness at the unfairness of this tragedy. There is usually nothing anyone did to cause, or could have done to prevent, a stillbirth. Yet, parents especially may feel guilt and blame themselves for the death of their baby. Parents may also experience feelings of loneliness and longing, helplessness, or, because of the intensity of their emotions, confusion.

These emotions are real and a normal part of grieving. Grieving is a process of making meaning out of the loss and of life without their baby. Grieving is not easy. It is long, unpredictable, and requires a lot of energy. Parents and family members need time to grieve since grieving is necessary to work through pain toward healing

A WOMAN'S STORY

"I was thrilled about being pregnant. After all I had gone through fertility treatment with my husband Steven to achieve this precious state. It was our first pregnancy and it had been problem-free. In the eighth month, everything was almost ready. The baby's room was ready and Steven was nearly done refinishing the cradle his mother had used to rock him as a baby. A few days before their next prenatal visit, I noticed that the baby had not moved for some time. I thought that the baby must have been sleeping. The next day I still did not feel the baby move. John told me everything was probably all right, but I sensed that something was wrong. I went to the doctor's office and the doctor could not find the baby's heartbeat and ultrasound confirmed what I had feared. Our baby was dead."

SUMMARIZING QUESTION & ANSWER

If Stillbirth Happens Once Will It Happen Again?

Extensive evaluation of the baby and placenta may help determine the chance that stillbirth could happen again. On average, there is approximately a 3% chance for stillbirth to recur in a next pregnancy—or approximately a 97% chance that a future pregnancy would not end in stillbirth. Finding a specific cause may imply a much higher or lower risk than this average one. In almost all circumstances, healthy pregnancies are possible.

What Can Friends and Family Do To Help at a time of Reproductive Loss?

Naturally, there is an urge to ease sorrow. Realistically, there is nothing anyone can say or do to take away their pain. You *can* provide love, hope, understanding, and the same support you would offer to anyone who has experienced the death of a loved one.

- Ignoring the subject does not make it go away nor does it make parents feel less pain. *Acknowledge the stillborn baby.* Most parents and family members need to talk about the death and about their baby. Use the baby's name or refer to "the baby" and let parents know that you are willing and interested in hearing about their experience if they wish to share it with you.

- *Acknowledge and validate the grief* parents and family members may feel following stillbirth. Help them by allowing and encouraging them to express their feelings and concerns.

- *Don't be silent* just because finding the "right" words to say is sometimes difficult. A simple "I've been thinking about you," "I'm sorry", or "I'm here if you would like to talk" can be comforting and reassuring.

- Sometimes presence is more powerful than words. Be there to provide a shoulder to lean on or a hand to hold. *Be there to listen.*

- *Let parents make their own decisions.* Encourage them to do what is best for them and support them in whatever they choose.

Your patience, love, and understanding are important immediately following the stillbirth and are also needed as time passes. Grieving takes time. Parents and family members will not be "done thinking about the baby" after a month or even a year. Their baby will never be forgotten. Continual love and support will help parents to work through their tragedy and cope with this painful experience. *You* can make a difference.

PART II

The How and Why of Miscarriage

4

Evaluation of Your Miscarriage

I. WHAT YOU MAY BE CONCERNED ABOUT

How common is miscarriage?

When considering this question, it is helpful to ask how often pregnancy occurs on average each cycle. Studies looking at very sensitive pregnancy tests suggest that pregnancy will occur in at least 60% of natural cycles in fertile couples.

The risk of miscarriage decreases as pregnancy progresses. It is possible that as many as 50% of pregnancies miscarry before implantation in the womb occurs. Early after implantation, pregnancy loss rate is about 30% (i.e. this is still before a pregnancy is clinically recognized). After a pregnancy may be clinically recognized (between days 35-50) about 25% will end in miscarriage. The risk of miscarriage decreases dramatically after the 8th week as the weeks go by.

Why did it happen—was it my fault?

When you conceive a baby, it takes half its genes from the sperm and half from the egg that ovulated that month. At the exact time of conception, the crossover of these genes takes place. Sometimes, genetic information is lost during this transfer process and the pregnancy is destined from that point not to be. It might be that this lost information is not needed for many weeks, and the pregnancy will continue as normal until that time. When the needed information is not there, it is then that the baby dies and you begin to miscarry. Sometimes when this happens, the miscarriage doesn't happen right away. This is called a *'missed'* miscarriage and may not be noticed until some weeks later.

These are the most common reasons that women miscarry. Miscarriage doesn't occur because of something you did or didn't do.

I've miscarried before—is it more than bad luck?

Perhaps…the probability of miscarriage is so common that it may occur more than once without representing any significant abnormality. Seeking a physician evaluation would be prudent in order to deliver if a reason may be detected and treatment rendered.

What is a recurrent miscarriage?

Recurrent miscarriage is diagnosed when a woman miscarries consecutively 3 times, before 20 weeks gestation. It is true that some women miscarry more often than chance alone would expect. When considering how common recurrent miscarriage actually is, we need to consider some numbers.

How common is recurrent miscarriage?

Many women miscarry more than once in their life. Considering the frequency of miscarriage, about 1 in 36 women will have 2 miscarriages due to nothing more than chance the risk of miscarriage related to one's pregnancy history may be summarized as follows:

Overall 15% of all clinically recognized pregnancies end in miscarriage. The main cause is a problem with the gene crossover at time of conception. This is due to chance alone, and nothing can be done to prevent it. When pregnancy is diagnosed much earlier, with very sensitive hormone tests, it is found in fact that up to 60% of pregnancies end in miscarriage—most would just present as a heavier late period if undiagnosed.

Considering this figure of 15%, we would expect only 0.4 % of women to miscarry 3 times consecutively, and it is due to nothing more than chance. In fact, 0.8-1.0% of women do so, suggesting other factors may be involved.

Other things that may contribute to early pregnancy loss include:

• Maternal age—there is a rise in miscarriage risk as maternal age increases. For women less than 35, the clinical miscarriage rate is 5-10%, for ages 35-40 it is 15-20% and over the age of 40 it is 25-30%.

- Diabetes that is poorly controlled—but not that which is well controlled

- Scleroderma—a soft tissue disease

- Smoking—30-50% increased risk

- Occupational exposure to solvents increases the risk of miscarriage

- Multiple pregnancy

What makes one prone to recurrent miscarriage?

- Medical disease—e.g. Systemic Lupus Erythematosus (SLE) which is a disease affecting many systems of the body. People affected often have a butterfly-rash over the cheeks and bridge of the nose.

- Antiphospholipid antibody syndrome—this is an immune disease where the main problems are RM, clots in the veins or arteries and often a low count of one of the blood components, called platelets.

- Chromosome problems—e.g. when egg and sperm unite, an unusual gene mismatch occurs.

- Uterine abnormality—e.g. a double-uterus or a septum down the middle. This is only associated in about 4% of recurrent miscarriage and is found in 1.8-3.6% of the normal population.

- Fibroids—circular clusters of uterine muscle growing within the uterine wall that may cause distortion of the uterine cavity.

- Cervical incompetence (weakness)—may cause miscarriage in 2nd trimester. This is more likely to be a cause of miscarriage if there is a history of surgery or trauma to the cervix.

- Polycystic ovary syndrome (PCOS)—this condition is a common cause of infertility due to the lack of ovulation, often associated with elevated androgens (male hormones). It has also been found when this is present with a raised hormone level (LH) there is an increased risk of miscarriage. Hormonal treatment for this is currently under investigation.

- Hormone deficiency—pregnancies that end in miscarriage may associate with low levels of a hormone called progesterone. This is thought to reflect an early pregnancy failure, and may be the result or the reason for the miscarriage.

- Immune problems—couples with recurrent miscarriage may have some similar components of the immune system. This is a controversial finding, under current investigation.

What Things are unlikely to cause recurrent miscarriage?

- Retroversion—or backward tilting of the uterus.

- Working when you're pregnant

- Exercise

- Sexual intercourse

- Air travel

- Not resting enough—bed rest doesn't alter whether you miscarry or not.

What investigations can be done?

The doctor will want to take a full history and examination looking for signs of the things mentioned above. Blood tests are taken to look for hormone irregularities or polycystic ovary syndrome (PCOS), SLE and Antiphospholipid syndrome, and so forth. Both partners may be checked for a chromosome (genetic) problem. An ultrasound scan may indicate the presence of PCOS. A HSG may detect structural uterine abnormalities. A hysteroscopy involves a tiny telescope look into the womb cavity to check for the presence of abnormalities or fibroids not seen on scan.

When can we start trying again?

Some couples decide that they want to begin trying for a pregnancy right away, while others feel that this is too soon and need time to get over this loss. There is no 'right' thing to do, and you have to go with your feelings.

We normally recommend that you wait one menstrual period after going home, and begin trying from then if you are emotionally ready. There is evidence that the risk of miscarriage in the next pregnancy is about 1.5 times higher if one menstrual cycle does not occur between two pregnancies.

What can I do to improve my chances for next time?

The most common reasons for miscarriage can't be helped; however you can prepare yourself for pregnancy. Taking in regular exercise, a healthy diet, reducing stress and getting your weight to within normal limits gives you something to concentrate on, and improves chances for long-term fertility. Certainly reducing your alcohol intake and stopping smoking will help, too. Remember to start taking folic acid to help normal development of the baby's nervous system.

What impact does a woman's age have on the frequency of miscarriage?

Female age has a very significant impact upon one's ability to achieve pregnancy and miscarriage. The older a woman and her eggs (that she was born with), the more likely there can be chromosomal mishaps, inevitable subfertility and miscarriage. Not all miscarriages are rooted in a chromosomal error. Therefore it is wise to request diagnostic studies to see if another reason for miscarriage may provide a therapeutic option.

When should I seek help?

You may choose to seek help and insight even after one miscarriage or difficulty in conceiving. Diagnostic studies may provide insight that can save valuable time as well as frustration, stress and grief.

Does stress cause a miscarriage?

Most doctors do feel that stress can reduce a woman's chance to conceive, but once pregnant, stress plays little role in miscarriage.

Will exercise cause a miscarriage?

Little information is available regarding the role and extent of exercise on pregnancy loss. It is felt that low-impact exercise is safe to perform in pregnancy.

Who should I see for help?

There are five types of medical doctors who can help you find a possible reason for miscarriage. The first is a Family Physician who can help order some of these basic tests. Then there are specialists in Obstetrics and Gynecology (OB/GYN), who may have already been part of your pregnancy care. Subspecialists of OB/GYN in a field called Reproductive Endocrinology tend to specialize in fertility related issues. Urologists may evaluate men for a cause of low sperm quality.

I had a D&C—will this cause any problems?

A D&C (dilatation and curettage) or evacuation is carried out to reduce the chance of infection and ensure that you don't continue bleeding over the following weeks. Very rarely, it can cause infection of the uterine lining or scar tissue within the uterine cavity. The chance of infection is less likely than had you not undergone a D&C. If this happens it usually responds well to a short course of antibiotics. The D&C doesn't weaken your cervix or make you more likely to miscarry in subsequent pregnancies.

How long will this bleeding last and when will my periods return?

Uterine bleeding may continue for about 7-10 days. Normally your next period will come by 6 weeks or so. If they were irregular before, then it may be longer. Also, your fertility returns before your next period, so if you feel pregnant again a pregnancy test might be useful.

What causes pregnancy loss?

Pregnancy losses comprise two major groups: chromosomally and/or morphologically abnormal and chromosomally and morphologically normal abortuses. Cytogenetic analysis has revealed that up to 60 percent of first-trimester losses and 30 to 40 percent of all recognized losses before 28 weeks involve abnormal karyotypes. Thus a relatively small proportion of all pregnancy loss occurs among embryos and fetuses that are chromosomally and morphologically normal. The reasons for the latter losses are not clear but may involve endocrine disorders, thyroid dysfunction, uterine abnormalities, cervical incompetence, maternal infections and other diseases, immunologic factors, environmental toxins, and psychogenic factors.

Am I too old—is it my age?

The only variable that appears to be consistently associated with miscarriage and infertility is age. Traditionally, female fertility was not thought to decline until after the age of 35. Fertility rates for population groups who do not practice contraception generally suggest that female fertility peaks around age 25 and then gradually declines. Studies have been able to eliminate the influence of many extraneous factors by studying conception rates after artificial insemination with frozen donor sperm in more than 2,000 nulliparous women whose husbands were azoospermic. The results of these studies suggest that the probability of conceiving declines noticeably at around age 30; the probability of success of insemination for 12 cycles was 73 percent for those 25 years and under, 74 percent for those 26 to 30, 61 percent for those 31 to 35, and 54 percent for those over 35. Population surveys from the United States and developing countries suggest that the risk of infertility increases steadily with female age, particularly after the age of 30. A specific reason for the decline in fertility years before the actual onset of menopause is the steady decline in egg quality with age. Endometriosis and the increasing risk of pelvic inflammatory disease with sexual exposure undoubtedly contribute to the overall increase in infertility with age.

The decline in fertility with the age of the women may also partially reflect an increase in early, unrecognized pregnancy loss. Chromosomal abnormalities, which make up a substantial proportion of abortuses, especially at early gestational ages, are known to rise with maternal age.

The overall rate of recognized pregnancy loss also increases with age. Women over the age of 35 have close to a twofold increased risk of spontaneous miscarriage compared to those under the age of 20. The increased risk of recognized miscarriages with maternal age is thought to be true for both chromosomally normal and abnormal conceptions.

Are there differences in miscarriage rates for different ethnic and socioeconomic groups?

Marked regional and ethnic variations in infertility have been observed and these variations have primarily been attributed to differential rates of infections of the reproductive organs. A 1976 survey in the United States showed that twice as many black couples as white couples were infertile, and that the racial differential was particularly high for couples when the wife was in the 20-to 24-year age group. Educational status exerted a lesser influence on infertility, but conception rates were lower among women who had not completed a high school education.

Socioeconomic class differences in spontaneous miscarriage rates and fetal deaths early and late in pregnancy are approximately twice as high for non-whites as for whites. Interrelationships between ethnic, racial and socioeconomic class differences in infertility and pregnancy loss have related to sexually transmitted diseases, nutritional status, prenatal care, and environmental exposures.

If I have miscarried before, what is my chance of miscarriage with my next pregnancy?

A link between previous spontaneous miscarriages and subsequent secondary infertility is suspected. The underlying mechanism for fertility impairment and the failure to maintain a pregnancy may be the same for some patients.

The risk of a subsequent spontaneous miscarriage has been shown to rise with the number of previous pregnancy losses. The risk of having a miscarriage in general is 15%. This risk increases to 24% after one miscarriage has occurred and rises to 35% after two miscarriages. The rate of miscarriage after three losses increases to 47%.

Number of Previous Miscarriages	Percent (%) of Repeat Miscarriages
No previous miscarriages	15%
1 previous miscarriage	24%
2 previous miscarriages	35%
3 previous miscarriages	47%

I had a miscarriage—did this cause me to miscarry now that I want to be pregnant?

Numerous studies have examined the impact of induced miscarriages on subsequent spontaneous miscarriage. There is no convincing evidence that a single induced miscarriage increases the risk of first-trimester losses. Rarely, scar tissue inside the uterine cavity from a pregnancy termination complication (e.g. Infection) may cause pregnancy loss. The effect of multiple induced miscarriages on subsequent pregnancy maintenance has not been determined.

Could a Sexually Transmitted Diseases Cause my Miscarriage?

Pelvic inflammatory disease (PID) represents the major cause of tubal obstruction leading to infertility. In the United States the annual incidence of PID has increased dramatically since 1960. Major sources of PID are gonorrhea and chlamydia, which may be responsible for more than 40 percent of cases. *Mycoplasma* organisms have been observed in women with gynecologic infections as well.

Syphilis represents an established cause of pregnancy loss. Although public health programs and the use of penicillin have reduced the impact of syphilis, this disease remains a serious health problem. Gonorrhea is not thought to cause pregnancy loss directly, but because PID may increase the risk of ectopic pregnancy these infections may indirectly contribute to pregnancy loss. Endometrial colonization of *Mycoplasma* organisms has been noted in a substantial proportion of habitual aborters. Although mycoplasma has been found more frequently in miscarriages, the exact relationship between these organisms and pregnancy loss has not been determined.

What role does nutrition play with my difficulty conceiving?

Severe dietary restrictions have been linked with lowered fertility. Food deprivation is thought to affect fertility primarily because of the decrease in ovulation during times of starvation. Voluntary dietary disturbances, as in the case of anorexia nervosa and bulimia, have also been associated with menstrual disturbances and cessation of ovulation.

Nutritional disturbances in the opposite direction, i.e., obesity, may also be associated with menstrual abnormalities. A retrospective survey found that women with prolonged and irregular cycles and reported hirsutism were significantly heavier than those who had regular menstrual cycles and no reported excess growth of facial hair. Furthermore, the occurrence of irregular and prolonged cycles was positively correlated with degree of obesity. In addition, women who had been obese as teenagers were more likely to be nulliparous. These findings suggest that excess fatty tissue may alter hormonal production and ovulation.

Can exercise have caused my miscarriage?

There is less of a consensus regarding the effect of moderate chronic malnutrition on fecundity. Frisch and Revelle originally set forth the hypothesis that the onset and maintenance of menstrual cycling in women is related to a threshold level of weight or body composition. This hypothesis, though not universally accepted, has stimulated extensive research on the role of diet and nutritional status in reproductive functioning. In addition to women suffering from severe nutritional deprivation, women athletes, particularly long-distance runners, and ballet dancers have been found to experience a high incidence of amenorrhea and anovulatory cycles. Although the menstrual disturbances among the latter groups have been correlated with reduction in weight or body fat, there is also some evidence that physical stress may independently affect circulating levels of reproductive hormones. Because normal menstrual cycles have been found to resume with weight gain and/or cessation of exercise, these generally represent temporary effects on fertility.

There is little information about the role of strenuous exercise on fetal loss. A Bulgarian study found no evidence of adverse pregnancy outcomes among its female Olympic athletes, despite the fact that some continued their training and even competition during the first months of pregnancy. Most professional athletes, however, probably tend to either stop training or restrict their activities once a pregnancy is recognized.

Can stress cause infertility or miscarriage?

Emotional factors are thought to play a significant role in infertility. Underlying psychopathology has also been linked to the induction of amenorrhea in the case of patients with anorexia nervosa. In addition to amenorrhea, emotional stress mediated by the hypothalamic-pituitary-gonadal axis may theoretically result in other ovulatory disorders such as luteal phase deficiency (progestational deficiency) and irregular ovulation.

Emotional factors have also been linked to pregnancy loss, particularly habitual miscarriage. In a study of habitual aborters and patients who had no history of spontaneous miscarriage, psychological tests revealed more emotional instability, tension, hostile feelings, and guilt in the former than the latter group. Others have similarly stated that habitual aborters tend to have marked psychic conflicts. Although psychotherapy has been reported to be successful in treating some habitual aborters, there is again no clear evidence that the psychological problems were the underlying cause of the pregnancy losses.

Does drinking alcohol and smoking contribute to miscarriage?

There are reports that cigarette smoking can be regarded as an etiologic risk factor for infertility. Smoking may interfere with tubal ciliary function with risks of ectopic tubal pregnancy higher in women who smoke. Cigarette smoking has been found to be a risk factor for spontaneous miscarriage in a few studies, but once adjustments were made for the effect of alcohol consumption only a weak association has been evident between smoking and pregnancy loss. A report from Utah suggested that households with a high caffeine intake had an increased risk of fetal loss.

Women drinking alcohol twice a week or more during pregnancy had more than a twofold increased risk of a spontaneous miscarriage than nondrinkers. In a prospective investigation women who had an average of one to two drinks daily were twice as likely to have a second-trimester loss than those who reported drinking no alcohol during early pregnancy. Whereas these investigators concluded that their data indicated that even moderate consumption of alcohol during pregnancy might be a risk factor for miscarriage, others have suggested that the increased risk is probably limited to the heaviest or most frequent drinkers.

Can drugs cause pregnancy loss?

Habitual use of barbiturates, narcotics, and tranquilizers has also been linked with menstrual abnormalities. Few controlled studies, however, have examined the effects of medications or illicit drugs on fertility. Mercury is also known to increase the rate of miscarriage. In general, little is known about the role of prescription, over-the-counter, or illegal drugs on pregnancy loss.

Uterine and tubal anomalies have been found in women exposed to diethylstilbestrol (DES) in *utero*. Although several studies have indicated that DES daughters may have reduced fertility and increased pregnancy loss, the role that the structural abnormalities play in reproductive impairment remains controversial.

What occupational or environmental exposures should I be worried about?

The growing participation of women in the labor force has led to considerable concern about possible hazards to reproduction from exposures in the work place. The unprecedented number of new and increasingly complex chemicals, which may pollute our air, water, and food, has also raised concern about the potential reproductive effects of environmental pollutants. Nevertheless, few controlled studies have been conducted to evaluate the effects of such exposures on female fertility or pregnancy maintenance.

Many of the substances that are suspected of lowering a woman's fertility are also thought to affect pregnancy loss. Women working in the pottery and white lead industry during the late nineteenth century were more likely to be sterile or, if they became pregnant, to miscarry than women who were not employed in lead work. The deleterious reproductive effects of chronic low-level occupational or environmental exposure to lead are less well established.

Carbon disulfide exposure among women in the textile industry has been reported to lead to menstrual disorders, decreased fertility, and excess fetal loss. Women working in rubber, leather, dry cleaning, and other industries where benzene was used as a solvent were historically at risk for chronic benzene poisoning. This condition, although not directly associated with infertility, might interfere with the ability to conceive and maintain a pregnancy. Increased spontaneous miscarriage rates have also been reported for female chemical workers, particularly those working in plastics, the pharmaceutical industries, and laundries, and for women occupationally exposed to ethylene oxide. Menstrual disorders have also been reported among women working in factories formulating oral contraceptives and among flight attendants. It is not clear whether the effect in the latter group reflects stress, irregular work schedules, or disruption of circadian rhythm, or such possibly hazardous exposures as increased ozone concentrations, although the former seems more probable.

Use of herbicides containing dioxin as a contaminant has prompted considerable concern over possible adverse effects, but there are no convincing data as yet that dioxin contaminants have affected reproduction. Toxic waste dumps, such as the Love Canal landfill in New York State, which contains more than 200 organic compounds including dioxin, benzene, and toluene, have also elicited widespread attention. An investigation of adverse pregnancy outcomes among women in the Love Canal area found only a slight increase in spontaneous miscarriages.

The widespread use of video display terminals in the home and in the work place have raised concerns regarding non-ionizing radiation emissions from these terminals. Spontaneous miscarriage clusters have been reported among female video display terminal operators, but these "clusters" are thought to represent random statistical events.

Can a man's age play a role in a women's miscarriage?

Paternal age is thought to affect fertility and pregnancy loss. Although the woman's age contributes directly to reproductive loss, the age of the father over age 50 has been found to contribute to the risk fetal chromosome abnormalities such as trisomy 21. The prevalence of certain autosomal dominant disorders, e.g., achondroplasia, has nevertheless been shown to rise with paternal age, even when corrected for maternal age.

What sexually transmitted diseases contribute to infertility?

Genital infections, if they are not treated properly, can lead to blocked sperm ducts and, as a result, abnormal spermatogenesis. Gonorrhea and Chlamydia infections represent major sources of urethritis and epididymitis in the developing and the developed worlds. *Mycoplasma* infections are also known to cause urethritis in the United States, but its etiologic role in male infertility has not been established.

It has been known for some time that mumps in postpubertal males may cause orchitis, which in turn can lead to sterility. The proportion of men with mumps who suffer fertility impairment is nevertheless estimated to be quite small. Febrile illnesses and certain diseases primarily found in developing countries, e.g., urogenital tuberculosis, filariasis, and leprosy, have also been implicated in male infertility.

What psychological factors affect a man's fertility?

The association between psychic stress and impotence is well established. Some have estimated that 90 percent of the cases of impotence may be psychogenic in origin. Others have cautioned that this may be an overestimate, as there is a tendency to ascribe impotence to psychic stress if no organic cause is found. Nevertheless, impotence probably represents the most common psychosexual disorder in men.

The importance of emotional factors in abnormal spermatogenesis is less well established. There are case reports of men whose sperm counts have dropped to azoospermic levels as a result of severe anxiety, tension, or trauma. Stress, in the form of every-day life experiences or adjustment difficulties, has been associated with a less severe effect on spermatogenesis. A study of subfecund marriages found that oligospermia was substantially higher among recent migrants than among nonrecent migrants or nonmigrants. The fact that spermatogenesis has been found to improve as psychic stress subsides provides further confirmation that the stress was the underlying etiologic factor. According to some authorities, however, psychic stress is not a common cause of clinical spermatogenic dysfunction.

Will alcohol consumption affect my ability to get pregnant?

Although there is no epidemiologic evidence that alcohol consumption affects male fertility, chronic alcohol abuse has been associated with hypogonadism, which in turn can lead to abnormal spermatogenesis, impotence, and gynecomastia. Moderate drinking is thought not to affect reproductive capacity in most men but may impair fertility in those with borderline sperm counts.

Does cigarette smoking affect male fertility?

There is conflicting evidence as to whether cigarette smoking affects male reproduction. Some investigators have concluded that cigarette smokers have more sperm abnormalities than nonsmokers. Semen quality has also been reported to improve in infertile men after they stopped smoking.

Do drugs affect male fertility?

Chemotherapy, sulfasalazine, which is used in the treatment of ulcerative colitis, and certain psychotropic drugs, may cause temporary or permanent sterility. A major constituent of marijuana, delta-9-tetrahydrocannabinol, is reported to have a modest, reversible suppressive effect on sperm count and motility.

Men who have been exposed to DES *in utero* have been found to have an increased incidence of a variety of genital tract abnormalities, including epididymal cysts, maldescended testes, hypoplastic testes, varicoceles, and spermatozoal defects. These findings suggest that DES exposure may result in reduced male fertility.

What environmental and occupational exposures are of concern?

Excess heat and exposure to certain chemical and physical agents may lower male fertility. A high scrotal temperature can impede sperm maturation. Suggested causes of elevated scrotal temperature are tight underclothing, frequent hot baths or sauna, and prolonged sitting. The effect of extreme heat on spermatogenesis is thought to be reversible in most cases.

One of the few occupational exposures that have clearly been shown to affect testicular function is dibromochloropropane (DBCP), a soil pesticide. Men employed in the manufacture as well as application of DBCP were found to have depressed sperm counts, with some of the factory workers demonstrating clinical infertility. Whether the sperm count depression is reversible is not clear. Manufacture of DBCP in the United States was discontinued after the toxic effects of this pesticide came to public attention. Ethylene dibromide, which replaced DBCP as a common pesticide, has been under suspicion as well, but to date there is no convincing evidence that it impairs male reproductive potential. Occupational exposure to kepone, as well as unspecified types of pesticides has also been reported to cause impotence and infertility.

Sperm abnormalities and sexual malfunction have been attributed to several other occupational exposures, including lead, chloroprene, carbon disulfide, and synthetic estrogens. It has even been hypothesized that the fall of Rome resulted from sterility in the ruling class caused by excess consumption of lead-contaminated wine. Irradiation can also alter sperm production, but its effect appears to be reversible in many cases. As is the case for women, there are no studies that show that *in utero* irradiation adversely affects subsequent fertility in men.

Paternal exposures have also been linked to spontaneous miscarriages, specifically occupational exposures to anesthetic gases, DBCP, vinyl chloride, dioxin contaminants (Agent Orange), and chloroprene. The available evidence for these effects is limited and conflicting, and further documentation is needed before the role of paternal occupational and environmental exposures in pregnancy loss can be established.

II. EVALUATION: HELP FROM YOUR DOCTOR—WHAT IS IMPORTANT TO KNOW...

Anatomical

- Malformation of uterus—e.g., T-shaped uterus or uterine septum
- Incompetent cervix
- Uterine fibroids
- Adhesions (scar tissue) inside uterus

Procedures to diagnose:

- Hysterosalpingogram
- Hysteroscopy
- Sonogram
- Laparoscopy

Hormonal

- Inadequate amount of progesterone—luteal phase defect
- Abnormal function of other hormone secreting organs, e.g., thyroid, adrenal, pituitary

Procedures to diagnose:

- Physical exam
- Ultrasound
- Blood hormone tests
- Basal body temperature graph

• Endometrial biopsy

Teratogens—agents that can interfere with normal fetal development

• Significant x-ray exposure

• Chemical exposure at work or at home

• Drug exposure—prescription and non-prescription

• Alcohol and substance abuse

• Infectious agents—rubella, toxoplasmosis, cytomegalovirus, herpes, mycoplasma

Procedures to diagnose:

• Report known exposure history to physician

• Blood tests for exposure to infectious agents

Maternal Factors

• Mothers with medical conditions such as diabetes mellitus, lupus, and seizure disorders may be more prone to pregnancy loss.

• Maternal infection with 1-mycoplasm

• Maternal age 35 years and older can increase risk of pregnancy loss.

Procedures:

• Accurate diagnosis of medical condition

• Careful monitoring of medications in future pregnancy

PATERNAL FACTORS

• Paternal infection with mycoplasma exposures

- Bacterial infection of prostate, epididymis and urethra

Procedures to diagnose:

- Semen analysis for white blood cells

- Semen culture

<u>*Immunologic*</u>

- Maternal immune system unable to protect fetus from rejection

Procedures to diagnose:

- Immunologic testing via serum and/or fetal tissue

<u>*Genetic/Chromosome Abnormality*</u>

- The majority (50%-60%) of early pregnancy loss (less than 12 weeks) is due to an abnormal chromosome composition.

- Change in chromosome number or individual chromosome constitution can increase risk for miscarriage.

- Occasionally inherited (from either parent) chromosome rearrangements pre-dispose one to a miscarriage.

Procedures following loss

- Blood chromosome testing (in cases of suspected inherited abnormalities)

<u>*Placenta & Cord*</u>

- Placenta abruption—premature separation of placenta

- Placenta previa—placenta is overlapping the cervix

- Placental infection

- Knot in umbilical cord

- Cord wrapped around fetus

Procedures to diagnose:

- Ultrasound exam of placenta and umbilical cord

Pre-term Labor

- Premature onset of labor (6-10% of all births are pre-term)

Procedures to prevent:

- Examination for general medical conditions

- Careful assessment of uterus, especially of cervix

Recurrent Pregnancy Loss Testing—A Case for Earlier Testing

Almost anyone who has suffered a miscarriage or stillbirth worries about the risk of having subsequent losses. Recent information indicates that women should look into recurrent pregnancy loss testing after two losses when it used to be common to wait until three. This is especially important for women in their 30s and 40s. Newer studies indicate a miscarriage rate of 26-40% after a woman has suffered two losses, so earlier testing makes sense emotionally, physically, and in many cases financially as well.

The tests and procedures listed below represent a mixture of the common elements of a recurrent pregnancy loss (RPL) evaluation and some of the more controversial immunological screenings. A doctor might choose to do any or all of them depending upon your unique history and needs.

Infection

- Mycoplasma

- Ureaplasma

- CMV

- Hepatitis B&C

- HIV

Some of these are infections that can be treated with antibiotics. Toxoplasmosis may be checked if you have cats in your house. Rubella immunity will also be tested and if non-immunity, you may receive a Rubella vaccine.

Thyroid

- Thyroid panel (TSH)

- Anti-Thyroid Antibodies

Thyroid problems can result in both fertility problems and miscarriage. If a problem is found, your physician will in many cases attempt to regulate the thyroid before another pregnancy is achieved.

Chromosomal

- Chromosome Testing on Fetal (Miscarriage) Tissue

    This can only be done right at the time of miscarriage. It is an analysis of the genetic makeup of the fetus. It can indicate genetic problems that lead to RPL. Many miscarriages are caused by chromosomal abnormalities that are unlikely to repeat. To know if the problem is likely to recur, it is necessary to study the genetics of both parents as well.

- Karyotyping of Parents

    Chromosome analysis of blood of both parents may show if there is a potential problem with one of the parents that leads to miscarriage. Karyotyping is often performed in conjunction with fetal testing to provide answers. These tests help rule out the 3% of partners that carry a chromosomal problem called a balanced translocation.

Anatomical

- Abdominal Ultrasound

• Transvaginal Ultrasound

The transducer uses sound waves to compute a picture of the baby, placenta and umbilical cord. It provides for a painless assessment of fetal anatomy in pregnancy.

• Hysterosalpingogram (HSG)

A hysterosalpingogram is where dye is injected into the uterus to look for anatomic problems, such as fibroids, polyps, scar tissue or structural problems with the uterine cavity, which are thought to cause about 15% of RPL. This test is usually done in the first half of a woman's cycle. A small catheter is inserted through the cervix in order to inject the dye while an x-ray is taken.

• Hysteroscopy

This is usually done under local or general anesthesia. Your cervix is dilated in order to insert a small fiberoptic scope in order to view the inside of your uterus. Abnormalities may be fixed during this procedure. This procedure is usually done under local or general anesthesia for comfort and to allow your doctor to sometimes perform this in conjunction with a laparoscopy.

• Laparoscopy

A laparoscopy is done to look for endometriosis, adhesions and malformations of the reproductive organs. The woman is usually under general anesthesia as carbon dioxide gas is used to expand the abdominal cavity to provide better viewing of the pelvic organs. The doctor will then insert a scope through a small incision made inside or just below the navel to view the outside of the uterus, ovaries and fallopian tubes. Often a second incision is made just below the pubic hairline through which an instrument is inserted to gently manipulate the organs to allow the scope to examine different angles. If found, endometriosis and adhesions may be removed during this surgery.

Luteal Phase Defect

A luteal phase deficiency is diagnosed when the length of time between ovulation and menses is under 12 days and/or the lining of the uterus does not develop enough to sustain a pregnancy.

- Endometrial Biopsy (EMB)

- Pelvic Ultrasound

The endometrial biopsy is used to "date" the lining to see if it is out of sync hormonally. It is considered out of phase if it the lining appears to be more than 2 days off. It is common to repeat the biopsy in another cycle; if it is found to be out of phase, before a diagnosis of a luteal phase defect is made.

The biopsy is performed in the second half of the cycle, usually just a few days before menstruation is expected. The biopsy is done by inserting a narrow catheter through the cervix and into the uterus. A small sample of tissue is sucked into the tube and sent to the lab for analysis. Expect a bit of discomfort with this test—about the same as a bad menstrual cramp. You may have some spotting afterward.

- Serum Progesterone Level

The serum progesterone level is a blood test measuring the progesterone produced by the corpus luteum. A good result is over 15 ng/ml.

Treatment:

A common treatment for a luteal phase problem is progesterone supplementation in the form of suppositories, injections, pills, or a combination of the above. The progesterone must be started at the time of conception (ovulation) in order to be useful. If started later, there is no statistical change in the rate of miscarriage.

Better ovulation may also be a solution for luteal phase deficiency. Enhancement of ovulation with agents such as clomiphene citrate, gonadotropins or HCG injections may also improve luteal phase deficiency.

Autoimmune

- Antiphospholipid Antibodies

- Anticardiolipin Antibodies

- Lupus Anticoagulant

• Anti-Nuclear Antibodies

Note that anti-Cardiolipin antibodies (ACA) are part of the group of anti-phospholipid antibodies (the other six are Phosphoethanolamine, Phosphoinositol, Phosphatidic acid, Phosphoglycerol, Phosphoserine, and Phosphocholine). It is fairly common to test for ACA, but a full work-up includes all seven anti-phospholipid antibodies being checked for three markers: IgG, IgA and IgM markers (so 21 different markers in all).

These tests diagnose a condition that can cause mainly 2nd trimester losses due to blood clots forming in the vascular system of the placenta. The condition is also responsible for some late 1st trimester losses.

This is the cause of about 10% or so of RPL. The treatment usually involves low-dose aspirin and heparin.

Alloimmune

• Natural "Killer Cells"

• Blocking Antibodies

The research in this area is fairly new and is very controversial. Laboratory variations in testing add to the confusion regarding efficacy of treatments and outcomes. Many physicians remain guarded regarding the role of this treatment for recurrent pregnancy loss.

Diabetes

• Blood Sugar

Blood work for diabetes, which can cause stillbirths, but probably does not contribute much (if any) to miscarriages.

Summary of Clinical Information for a Women with Recurrent Pregnancy Loss

History

    Previous pregnancy outcomes

Diethylstilbestrol (DES) exposure

Menstrual pattern

General medical problems

Use of cigarettes or alcohol

Occupational history

Environmental exposure

Physical Examination

Abnormalities of Reproductive Organs

Uterine anomalies

Cervical changes (i.e. DES-related)

Thyromegaly

Galactorrhea

Evidence of infection

Evidence of systemic disease

Laboratory Evaluation

Complete blood count

Activated partial thromboplastin time (PTT)

Antinuclear antibody (ANA)

Anticardiolipin antibody (ACL)

Antiphospholipid antibody (APL)

Prolactin

Thyroid-stimulating hormone

Cervical cultures

Endometrial biopsy

Radiologic Work-up

Hysterosalpingogram

Sonohysterogram

Intravenous pyelogram or ultrasound (as indicated)

Surgery (as indicated)

Hysteroscopy

Laparoscopy

Chromosomal Evaluation

Peripheral karyotype—male and female

Cytogenetics of products of conception

CONCLUSION

Although the preceding discussion has focused on female and male factors separately, it is important to emphasize that reproductive failure can be a multifactorial disorder involving both female and male factors. Many of these factors may be acting independently of each other, but some may produce effects only in the presence of others. This review also underscores the need for epidemiologic research on infertility. It has been suggested that gene mutations may be responsible for no more than 10 percent of infertility. Presumably, environmental influences account for a sizable proportion of the remaining cases of infertility. Yet only a few correlates of female or male infertility have been identified. Apart from maternal age, sexually transmitted diseases, significant dietary disturbances, psychic stress, certain toxic drug treatments, and possibly *in utero* exposure to DES, the available evidence for any other risk factors of female infertility, e.g., tobacco, alcohol, or occupational exposures is at best suggestive. The list of factors that have been documented as being associated with male sexual malfunction or inadequate spermatogenesis is even shorter: sexually transmitted infections and other diseases; emotional disturbances; occupational exposure to DBCP, certain drug therapies, and possibly chronic alcohol abuse. Furthermore, only a few of these factors, e.g., sexually transmitted diseases, may be of major epidemiologic importance in either female or male infertility.

Although random genetic or developmental abnormalities of the embryo may be responsible for a substantial proportion of pregnancy losses, environmental factors are suspected of being associated with both genetically abnormal and normal miscarriages. Despite the more extensive epidemiologic research on pregnancy loss, the findings have generally been disappointing. Advanced maternal age, a history of pregnancy loss, and maternal infections and illnesses are among the few important epidemiologic predictors of spontaneous miscarriages. Certain drug therapies have been found to cause fetal death, but such therapies are uncommon among pregnant women. The effect of high-dose radiation on pregnancy outcome has been difficult to document in humans, and such exposure probably represents a rare cause of embryonic or fetal death. More evidence is needed before *in utero* exposure to DES can clearly be implicated in subsequent pregnancy loss. Only a weak association has been suggested between cigarette smoking and fetal loss, and the role of alcohol consumption in pregnancy loss awaits confirmation. The reproductive effects of maternal or paternal occupational exposures to anesthesia or other agents in the work place today are similarly open to question.

Although considerable progress has been made in identifying the mechanisms responsible for reproductive failure, much remains to be learned regarding the epidemiologic factors associated with infertility and early pregnancy loss.

III. CASE HISTORY

Mary B. presented as a 41-year-old woman with a 3 year old child and three subsequent miscarriages. She had no difficulty conceiving, in fact she would conceive rather quickly, but would miscarry at approximately 8 weeks. Her history was significant for her son being delivered by cesarean section for breech presentation.

A Hysterosalpingogram (HSG) was ordered and there was an area of the uterine cavity that did not completely fill with dye. She was advised to have a Hysteroscopy as an outpatient and intrauterine scar tissue was confirmed and treated at the same operative event. She subsequently conceived and surpassed the 12th week of pregnancy and delivered a full term baby without any problems.

5

The Biologic Clock—Impact of a Women's Age

REPRODUCTION AND AGE

AGE AND EGG QUALITY: LOWER FERTILITY AND HIGHER MISCARRIAGE

Pregnancy rates decrease between the ages of 35 and 40, and then drop off markedly after age 40. Miscarriage rates of IVF-ET pregnancies increase steadily with age, from 18% at ages 25-29, to 29% at age 40. Figure 1 demonstrates the impact of age on fertility:

FIGURE 1

Impact of Female Age on Fertility Outcome

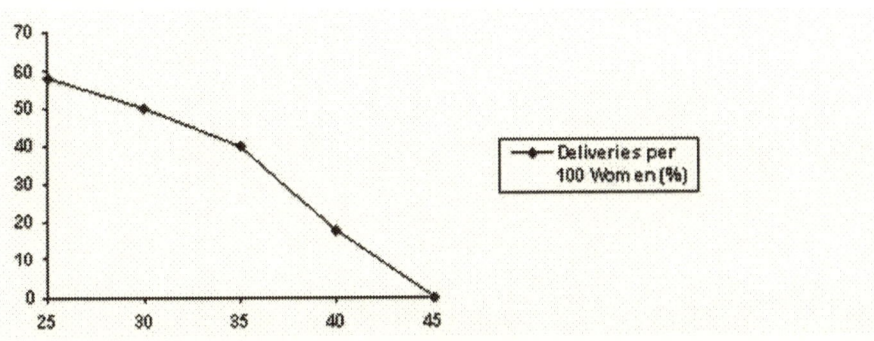

A direct relationship exists between a woman's age and miscarriage: the older a woman is, the higher her likelihood of miscarriage. Conversely, the younger a woman is the less likely she is to miscarry.

ANATOMY OF THE EGG: ZONA PELLUCIDA

The outer wall of the egg is known as the Zona Pellucida. This Zona plays a vital role in allowing one sperm and only one sperm to enter the egg and hence successfully fertilize. Studies have shown that this wall thickens with age, therefore adding a considerable barrier to sperm penetration and fertilization, which may have existed when the woman was younger and the Zona thinner.

The Zona also provides a significant deterrent to successful embryo implantation. One of the physical events that occur prior to embryo implantation is the process known as "hatching". Hatching is a process in which the embryonic cells leave the protective "shell" of the zona and attach to the endometrium to achieve a successful pregnancy.

CHROMOSOMES AND THE EGG

During an eggs final division into 23 chromosomes, the chromosomes line up in a vertical line. Along this line each pair splits down the middle and is pulled to the opposing side of the egg. In this manner an egg reduces its chromosome count in half—awaiting the other "half" of chromosomes to enter from the sperm.

As eggs age, it is postulated that the arms of the chromosomes get "sticky" and do not always go to their respective side. In this manner one set of chromosomes may be lacking a segment (monosomy) or one set of chromosomes may be in surplus a chromosome segment (trisomy), both of which are associated with miscarriage.

EGG DONATION

With good nutrition, exercise and avoidance of adverse lifestyle habits such as smoking, women are in better physical condition to maintain a pregnancy. Unfortunately, these attributes still don't assist the impact of a woman's chronologic age upon her ability to successfully conceive and maintain a pregnancy.

As a significant number of women enter the advanced reproductive years of 35-45 we see a need for an increasing array of options that includes egg donation. Egg donation is particular helpful for the woman who has poor egg quality as indicated in prognostic screening tests or a history of repeat reproductive losses.

6

Genetic Factors Associated with Miscarriage

A great number of early pregnancy losses represent genetically abnormal embryos that are formed from abnormal gametes that arise randomly during gametogenesis. Indeed, many miscarriages are never detected clinically and are not included in the earlier literature on recurrent miscarriage. Our understanding of pregnancy loss has increased from the experience gained from IVF. For example, we are very conscious of the fact that age is a significant factor in determining the eventual fate of a newly developed conceptus. As demonstrated by data from IVF programs treating women 40 years and older, there is a 50% spontaneous miscarriage rate in this age group, whereas there is about a 30% rate among younger women. Of the abnormal karyotypes, 44% to 60% exhibit trisomy (three chromosomes) and 18% to 24% exhibit Monosomy (one chromosome). Another 14% to 22% show polyploidy (three sets of chromosomes), and 4.5% have a structural basis

Genetic Factors

Between 50% and 60% of first trimester spontaneous miscarriages show evidence of genetic defects; the most common is trisomy (one extra chromosome), followed by X monosomy (one x-chromosome missing) and polyploidy (more than one extra chromosome). Of the familial translocations, about 66% are, maternally derived and the remainder is of paternal origin. Approximately 50% of all unbalanced translocations arise *de novo* or spontaneously during gametogenesis. The risk of delivering a live fetus with trisomy 21 is 10% to 15% if the mother carries the anomaly and 2% for a paternal carrier; approximately 50% of these conceptions will be lost to spontaneous miscarriage. The birth of a trisomy infant increases the risk of a subsequent trisomy pregnancy by 1%.

Abnormalities caused by single gene mutations (Mendelian disorders) or mutations at several loci (polygenic or multi-factorial disorders) cannot be detected by karyotype analysis. However, the future use of techniques such as florescence in situ hybridization (FISH) can identify these defects.

Work has only just begun on molecular mechanisms (e.g., structure and function of cell adhesion molecules and proteins involved in immune responses) that may be responsible for recurrent pregnancy loss.

CHROMOSOMAL ANALYSIS OF GAMETES AND EMBRYOS

A consensus of reports concerning aneuploidy rates in sperm indicates that about 0.1% of sperm are aneuploid. Few data about the cytogenetics of the human egg had been available prior to the expansion of IVF. Now that access to the human egg is available, genetic analyses have been performed demonstrating 26% of oocytes recovered after superovulation carry chromosomal abnormalities, mainly monosomies and trisomies. This rate appeared to be higher in older women (24% in the <35 versus 44% in the >35 age groups). An explanation for why age may influence the probability of a chromosomal defect is understood when considering the time course of ovum gametogenesis. Oocytes are "arrested" during meiosis for years, if not decades, prior to puberty and fertilization presents an egg's vulnerability to potential insult and genetic errors.

The first reported genetic analysis of human pre-embryos presented two out of three as chromosomally abnormal when karyotyped. Karyotyped human embryos at the two-to eight-cell stage, which appeared healthy, were abnormal 11% of the time and 19% of fragmented embryos were found to be chromosomally abnormal. Overall, 23% of embryos fertilized in vitro had a chromosomal abnormality.

Pregnancy Loss

The true rate of spontaneous early pregnancy loss in women postulated to be 78%. Three major studies have evaluated early pregnancy loss by using sensitive assays for HCG in the luteal phase of fertile women trying to conceive. Biochemical evidence of pregnancy was present at a 31% pregnancy rate per cycle. However, only 20% of cycles resulted in a clinical pregnancy, and a significant number of these were subsequently lost. Overall, 42% of all detected pregnancies resulted in a loss. If the clinical definition of recurrent miscarriage were applied to these pregnancies, the number of patients meeting these criteria would increase dramatically. However, evaluation subsequent cycles of these same couples demonstrates many of these patients to be highly fertile, with 30% conceiving in the next cycle following a reproductive loss, and 95% conceiving within a year. Clearly, these subclinical losses do not meet the classical criteria of recurrent pregnancy loss. In fact, this group of patients may have increased fertility. Calculation of the ongoing pregnancy rate per cycle from the summarized data yields an 18% ongoing pregnancy rate per cycle.

The most common pathologic finding in early spontaneous miscarriages is a developmental abnormality in the embryo or placenta. One of the leading causes of spontaneous miscarriages is a degenerated or "blighted ovum". The conceptus in an early miscarriage was significantly more likely to have a cytogenetic abnormality. Approximately 50% of miscarriages exhibit a chromosomal defect, with trisomies as a group being most common. Many trisomies observed in spontaneous miscarriages have never been found in live born offspring. This indicates that many of these chromosomal abnormalities are incompatible with life. Monosomy X is the most common single genetic defect that causes miscarriage.

Karyotype analysis has been performed on aborted material from an IVF program. Cytogenetic analysis was available in spontaneous miscarriages from pregnancies achieved by IVF. The rate of aneuploidy was found to be 38% with consensus that the risk of chromomosomal abnormalities in pregnancies achieved by IVF is lower than in spontaneous conceptions. This data supports the finding that the rate of aneuploidy in babies conceived by IVF is lower than in spontaneously achieved pregnancies (0.3% versus 0.6%).

GENETIC CAUSES OF RECURRENT PREGNANCY LOSS

The vast majority of miscarriages represent the manifestation of chromosomal abnormalities. Structural and numerical chromosomal abnormalities include translocations and inversions. Numerical chromosomal abnormalities include mosaicism.

A. Translocations

Translocations account for the greatest incidence of structural chromosomal abnormalities in recurrent miscarriages. Crossover or break and exchange of chromatin between any two nonhomologous (different) chromosomes during meiosis may result in a reciprocal translocation. This process may occur without loss of genetic material (i.e., total chromosome number is 46) and is then known as a balanced translocation. Individuals with a balanced translocation, although phenotypically normal, are predisposed to abnormal offspring with chromosomal imbalance. When the translocation is unbalanced, phenotypic abnormalities result. A variety of chromosomal abnormalities may result in the conceptuses of balanced translocation carriers depending upon the segregation of gametes at meiosis. Gametes often contain genetic excesses and deficiencies, resulting in zygotes that have partial monosomy and trisomy. Clinically, this may be manifested as a spontaneous miscarriage or the birth of a child with birth defects and retardation.

If a translocation involves homologous (same) chromosomes, known as a Robertsonian translocation, the prognosis is dismal. The only live born resulting from t(13;13) or t(21;21) is cytogenetically abnormal (trisomies 13 and 21, respectively); the other conceptions from these patients are monosomies 13 and 21, respectively, and terminate in spontaneous miscarriage. Women with such Robertsonian translocations should be informed about sterilization and assisted reproduction with donor eggs. Partners of male carriers should use donor sperm.

Of the 4% to 6% couples with recurrent pregnancy loss due to translocations, approximately 65% have reciprocal and 35% have Robertsonian translocations. In a study of over 5400 couples in which women with two or more spontaneous miscarriages were studied, the probability of one member of a couple to be a carrier increased with the number of miscarriages at the time of assessment. Survival of offspring with unbalanced chromosomes correlated with a minimum imbalance. The risk of clinically apparent spontaneous miscarriages for carriers of reciprocal translocations has been estimated to be as high as 50%. For carriers of Robertsonian translocations, the rate of clinically apparent spontaneous miscarriages has been reported to be less than 25%.

A review of the literature reveals half of the cases of unbalanced translocation in abortuses to be of genetic origin, whereas the other half arise spontaneously (de novo). These findings underline the uncertainty of assuming that translocations detected in abortuses indicate the presence of parental translocation.

Cytogenetic studies on couples whose reproductive history included one or more first-trimester spontaneous miscarriages have been performed to determine the frequency of parental translocations. They found that balanced chromosomal translocations have a very low occurrence (less than 0.4%) among couples having repeated spontaneous miscarriages without other abnormal pregnancies. Only women who had spontaneous miscarriages in addition to other abnormal perinatal events, including an anomalous live born infant, a stillborn infant, or an unexplained neonatal death, had an increased frequency of translocations. The association between frequency of translocations and number of prior miscarriages has yet to be clarified. A review of the combined data suggests that couples with four losses have a higher frequency of translocations than couples with fewer losses.

A "risk profile" may be formulated for each carrier of a balanced chromosome rearrangement that considers reproductive history, type of rearrangement, size of the imbalance, and sex of the trait carrier. In practice, however, cytogenetic studies presently remain the only truly effective means of assessing a couple's risk for a balanced translocation. In addition to genetic counseling, other family members should be karyotyped for the presence of the same translocation. The reproductive options for translocation carriers who wish to minimize the risk of abnormal offspring in a pregnancy include prenatal testing (i.e., chorionic villus sampling or amniocentesis), donor insemination for male carriers, and donor ova and IVF for female carriers. It is emphasized that prenatal screening is only appropriate after demonstration of at least one parental balanced translocation chromosomal rearrangement. There are no data supporting a recommendation that prenatal diagnosis be performed solely on the basis of recurrent spontaneous miscarriage without previous parental chromosomal analysis.

B. Inversions

Inversions result when two breaks occur in a chromosome and the intervening chromatin is inverted 180 degrees relative to the remaining chromatin and thereby reinserted in a reverse sequence. When this event involves only one arm (p or q) of the chromosome, it is referred to as a paracentric inversion. When the intervening piece includes the centromere, and thus a break in each arm (p and q), it is referred to as a pericentric inversion. Pericentric inversions may change the position of the centromere as well as the lengths of the chromosome arms and thus are more likely to be detected than paracentric inversions.

Inversions, as described, usually do not result in chromosomal imbalance and generally do not result in phenotypic abnormalities. Occasionally, a gene will be damaged or gene sequences may be altered, causing an altered expression of its new neighbor genes by a "position effect". Inversions result in the production of abnormal chromosomes during meiotic crossing over. This is in contrast to the situation of balanced translocations in which abnormal offspring result from chromosomal segregation at meiosis. The actual risk of abnormal offspring for inversion carriers based upon pooled empirical data derived from amniocentesis registries is 8% if the carrier is female and 4% if male. The higher risk associated with women is related to higher recombination frequencies noted in women than in men. Abnormal liveborns are more likely to occur if the inversion involves at least 50% of the chromosome.

Few paracentric inversions have been reported in couples with a history of recurrent miscarriages. Reproductive outcomes of paracentric inversion carriers are generally positive, with a relatively small risk of pregnancy loss.

Not all pericentric inversions are associated with the 4% to 8% risk of an abnormal liveborn, as previously mentioned. Pericentric inversions of chromosome 9 are the most commonly reported inversions in couples with recurrent miscarriages. However, the reported incidence of pericentric inversions of chromosome 9 in the general population (1.2%) approximates its reported incidence in couples with recurrent miscarriage. Thus, inversion of this small heterochromatic segment of chromosome 9 is considered to be a normal variant and probably does not contribute to recurrent miscarriages.

C. Mosaicism

Translocations represent structural rearrangements; mosaicism is an example of a numerical chromosomal abnormality. Mosaicism is the presence of two or more cell lines in the same individual with these cell lines arising from a single zygote or embryo from nondysjunction or anaphase lag. Nondysjunction occurs when both chromosomes of a homologous pair migrate to the same cell, resulting in cell lines with 45 and 47 chromosomes, respectively. If the X chromosome is involved, this will result in 45,X and 47,XXX lines. Anaphase lag occurs when one chromosome fails to segregate into either of the two daughter cells, resulting in 45,X and 46,XX lines if the X chromosome is involved.

The most common form of a sex chromosomal mosaicism is 45,X/46,XX. In a chromosomal study of 500 couples with two or more miscarriages, almost half of all abnormal karyotypes were mosaics. The majority of mosaicism occurred in the maternal X chromosome. In this study, maternal X-chromosomal mosaicism occurred as frequently as balanced parental translocation. The high prevalence of mosaicism found in couples with recurrent miscarriages underlines the importance of seeking mosaicism in these couples.

Monosomy X often presents as a mosaic. Pure monosomy X (45,X) is observed in about 10% of chromosomally abnormal abortuses. Although monosomy X is the single most common complement among abortuses, only 1 in 10,000 offspring that are liveborn have this lesion. In addition, patients with monosomy X manifest relatively few life threatening anomalies. Because approximately 2% of all conceptions are 45,X, 99% must be lost.

Polyploidy accounts for approximately 10% of recognized spontaneous miscarriages in the first trimester. Although triploidy occurs most often, tetraploidy has also been observed. The placenta of triploid fetuses may show hydropic changes. Tetraploid embryos cease development 2 to 3 weeks after fertilization, with no recognizable embryonic differentiation observed.

CHROMOSOMAL STRUCTURAL REARRANGEMENTS IN PARENTS

Chromosomal structural rearrangements, including deletions, duplications, inversions, and translocation, are associated with recurrent pregnancy loss and occur in 0.3% of the general population. In patients with an otherwise normal evaluation for spontaneous miscarriage, chromosomal evaluation is an important diagnostic tool in attempting to elicit a possible genetic cause.

The incidence of structural abnormalities in couples referred for evaluation of repetitive pregnancy loss has been estimated to be 5%. Balanced translocations are the genetic anomaly most commonly associated with recurrent fetal loss. Reciprocal and robertsonian translocations are the types most commonly associated with reproductive loss.

Patients with recurrent fetal loss and a documented chromosomal abnormality in one or both partners will have one of the following pregnancy outcomes: a spontaneous miscarriage, a normal live born infant, an infant with a balanced translocation, or an infant with an unbalanced translocation. The incidence of these outcomes has been documented in several studies involving patients with known chromosomal abnormalities. Evaluation of couples with chromosomal rearrangements and a history of recurrent spontaneous miscarriages will subsequently attempted to conceive and experience normal pregnancy outcomes 57%

of the time. Couples with reciprocal translocations who had been referred for two or more spontaneous miscarriages were successful in having a live-born infant over half of the time. Of the live born infants, 48% were of normal karyotype, 48% had a balanced translocation, and 4% had an unbalanced translocation.

The overall risk of detecting a fetal unbalanced karyotype in a mother with a balanced translocation and a history of recurrent miscarriages is 3.8%. These data emphasize the importance of prenatal diagnosis in parents with known chromosomal abnormalities.

Several methods are available for identifying chromosomal abnormalities in pregnancies. These include chorionic villus sampling (CVS) and amniocentesis. Chorionic villus sampling involves transcervical biopsy of trophoblastic tissue between the 9th and 12th weeks of gestation. A recent study on CVS reported a 99.6% success rate for obtaining cytogenetic results; no diagnostic errors were observed. Amniocentesis is an alternative means of fetal cytogenetic evaluation and is performed at approximately 16 weeks of gestation. The obvious advantage of CVS over amniocentesis is the opportunity for earlier diagnosis and intervention. The incidence of fetal loss is approximately 1.5% following amniocentesis and 3% following CVS. These procedures provide relatively safe and accurate means of prenatal diagnosis.

Summary

Pregnancy loss is a common finding when patients are monitored for biochemical signs of pregnancy early in gestation. Approximately 42% of pregnancies achieved do not reach viability. Chromosomal aberrations account for about 50% of cases of pregnancy loss when evaluated for aneuploidy. It is possible that a significant portion of euploid abortuses occur from undetectable (by present means) single gene defects. Genetic analysis of eggs and sperm provides some insight into mechanisms whereby approximately 30% of embryos generated are chromosomally abnormal.

Chromosomal aberrations cause recurrent pregnancy loss in a small number of instances. The three main causes are translocation, inversion, and mosaicism. Cells that result from division of progenitor cells containing these defects are at risk for aneuploidy. Translocations account for the greatest incidence of structural chromosomal abnormalities in recurrent miscarriages. Of the 4% to 6% of couples with recurrent pregnancy loss due to translocations, approximately 65% have reciprocal and 35% have Robertsonian translocations. Inversions cause pregnancy loss through unequal crossover between inversion loops. Mosaicism represents a numerical chromosome abnormality in which two cytogenetically different cell lines coexist. This imbalance is a cause of miscarriage.

Treatment of couples with recurrent spontaneous miscarriage requires cytogenetic analysis. Although many lesions are not treatable, their identification is required for optimal management. In the case of a Robertsonian translocation involving homologous chromosomes as described previously, offspring will be trisomy 13, trisomy 21, or a monosomy that results in spontaneous miscarriage. Donor gametes are required to treat these couples optimally. Other lesions require careful prenatal diagnosis with genetic counseling. Specific therapy for chromosomal causes of recurrent miscarriage requires a more complete understanding of the mechanisms whereby pregnancy loss occurs.

7

Environmental & Occupational Influences for Miscarriage

Environmental Toxins and Recurrent Pregnancy Loss

Toxic agents are a particularly important cause of pregnancy loss because exposure to them is so often preventable. Drugs and environmental agents may produce a variety of adverse effects that may be manifested together or independently. In a pregnant woman, these include maternal toxicity of many different kinds, teratogenesis, and the production of miscarriage.

A teratogen is an agent that can produce a permanent abnormality of structure or function in an organism that is exposed during embryonic or fetal life. An abortifacient is an agent that causes miscarriage. Most abortifacients seem to act by producing death of the embryo or fetus, but some abortifacients interfere with implantation or cause expulsion of the embryo from the uterus. Many teratogens are abortifacients, but some agents have only a teratogenic effect and others have only an abortifacient effect.

Embryonic or fetal death is often part of the spectrum of teratogenesis. Prior to implantation and before differentiation, the embryo is considered to be relatively resistant to the effects of teratogens, although it may be killed by a sufficiently toxic exposure. During organogenesis, moderate doses of teratogens are capable of inducing malformations, often in association with some embryonic death. Increasingly higher doses lead exclusively to embryonic death.

This is well illustrated by the effects of ionizing radiation in experimental animals. During the preimplantation stage, the embryo is insensitive to the teratogenic effects of radiation but is maximally sensitive to the lethal effects. The embryo becomes sensitive to the teratogenic effects but less sensitive to the lethal effects of radiation during organogenesis. Following the completion of organogenesis, malformations cannot be induced in the fetus, although the central nervous system remains sensitive to the teratogenic effects of radiation.

81

This example also emphasizes the importance of both gestational timing and dose on the effect produced by an environmental agent on the embryo or fetus. It is not possible to speak of an agent as an abortifacient without consideration of dose. Almost any agent that produces serious maternal systemic toxicity may be dangerous to the embryo or fetus. An agent that is generally considered to be safe, such as aspirin, may represent a serious hazard to the fetus if taken in a life-threatening overdose.

An environmental toxin can produce embryonic or fetal death in two entirely different ways. The first is by acting on the developing embryo or fetus itself during gestation. Only exposures of the pregnant woman are relevant in this regard. A second mechanism is by causing a genetic or chromosomal mutation in the gamete that, after fertilization, produces a lethal phenotype in the embryo or fetus.

The pharmacology of an agent in the adult is not a reliable predictor of its effect on the embryo or fetus. One cannot assume that an agent that produces a toxic effect in exposed individuals (i.e. a skin rash) is necessarily dangerous to the fetus. Conversely, a substance that has a low level of toxicity for adults may nevertheless be very hazardous to the embryo. Thalidomide provides a striking example of this. As an increasing number of women enter nontraditional jobs, there is growing concern that occupational exposures that are considered to be safe for an adult may not necessarily be safe for the embryo or fetus.

ENVIRONMENTAL FACTORS

Tobacco and Alcohol Exposure

It is estimated that 30% of reproductive-aged women smoke. Any history of smoking is associated with a 1.0 to 1.8 relative risk for miscarriage. The proposed mechanisms for tobacco-induced pregnancy loss include oxygen starvation. An impairment of fertility is created by a decrease in the function of the fallopian tubes, fertilization, embryonic cleavage and implantation by the toxins created by tobacco. Cigarette smoking has not been associated with birth defects. Smoking is a complex behavior associated with many other possibly confounding factors such as stress and malnutrition.

Alcohol

Alcohol, the most important human teratogen, causes a characteristic pattern of craniofacial, limb, and cardiovascular abnormalities known as the "fetal alcohol syndrome. This pattern of anomalies is typically seen among the children of women who drink heavily throughout pregnancy. Less severe anomalies may be seen with lower levels of alcohol consumption. Drinking during the first or second trimester of pregnancy has also been associated with an increased risk of miscarriage in a dose-dependent fashion.

No safe level for maternal drinking during pregnancy has been established. The combined effect of cigarette smoking and drinking during pregnancy appears to increase the rate of miscarriage compared to the effects of either agent alone.

A retrospective investigation in New York City reported that women drinking alcohol twice a week or more during pregnancy had more than twice the risk of a spontaneous miscarriage than nondrinkers. In a prospective investigation from California, women who had an average of one to two drinks daily were twice as likely to have a second-trimester loss, and those who consumed three or more drinks per day were more than three times as likely to miscarry during the second trimester than those who reported drinking no alcohol during early pregnancy.

Alcohol, Tobacco and Male Fertility

Although there is no epidemiologic evidence that alcohol consumption affects male fertility, chronic alcohol abuse has been associated with hypogonadism, which in turn can lead to abnormal spermatogenesis, impotence, and gynecomastia. Moderate drinking is thought not to affect reproductive capacity in most men but may impair fertility in those with borderline sperm counts. Some investigators have concluded that cigarette smokers have more sperm abnormalities than nonsmokers. Semen quality has also been reported to improve in infertile men after they stopped smoking.

Electromagnetic Fields

Exposure to electromagnetic radiation, such as that from video display units (VDUs), has been suggested to increase the risk of spontaneous pregnancy loss. Concern over the possibility that exposure to VDUs may be associated with miscarriage was prompted by the observation of several small clusters of adverse pregnancy outcome among women who worked with VDUs. In view of the millions of women who use VDUs daily and the frequency of miscarriage among the general population, many small clusters of this sort would be expected to occur by chance. Several large epidemiologic investigations of miscarriage among VDU users have been reported and no consistent association has been observed. Measurements have demonstrated that radiation emissions from VDUs are very low, often being less than background levels and invariably of a magnitude that is very unlikely to have any biologic effect. These findings suggest that use of VDUs by pregnant women is unlikely to pose any substantial risk of miscarriage.

Radiation.

Maternal exposure to ionizing radiation during pregnancy can produce malformations, fetal growth retardation, and embryonic death. In experimental animals, all of these effects show a dose-response relationship. The absorbed dose and rate of exposure as well as the stage of gestation determine which outcomes are most likely to be observed in a given instance. There is no indication that doses of radiation that typically occur with diagnostic studies pose a substantial risk of causing miscarriage, but data on this point are limited.

DRUGS

Chemotherapy, sulfasalazine, which is used in the treatment of ulcerative colitis and certain psychotropic drugs, may cause temporary or permanent sterility. Impotence has been reported among heroin and morphine addicts, and ejaculatory disorders have been cited as a possible side effect of tranquilizers and antihypertensive agents. However, a major constituent of marijuana, delta-9-tetrahydrocannabinol, is reported to have a modest suppressive effect on sperm count and motility.

Prescription and Non-Prescription Drugs

Case reports suggest that treatment during pregnancy with folic acid antagonists and such anticoagulants as warfarin can lead to fetal death. In general, little is known about the role of prescription, over-the-counter, or illegal drugs on pregnancy loss.

Cancer Treatments

Anti-cancer agents include alkylating agents such as cyclophosphamide, antimetabolites such as fluorouracil, and toxic antibiotics such as doxorubicin. Many anti-cancer agents have been found to produce malformations and fetal death in animals. A case-control study of 124 miscarriages among nurses found an association with occupational exposure to antineoplastic agents during the first trimester of pregnancy. This finding is not supported by clinical experience in pregnancies of women treated with much higher doses of antineoplastic drugs while receiving therapy for cancer.

DES

DES, diethylstilbestrol, is a drug that was given to millions of pregnant women, primarily from 1938 to 1971. This synthetic hormone was touted as a "wonder drug" and widely prescribed in the mistaken belief that it could prevent miscarriage. In addition to having no effect on miscarriage, it has resulted in health problems for the women who took the drug as well as their daughters and sons.

Women who have been exposed to DES *in utero* have been found to have an increased incidence of a variety of genital tract abnormalities, including a T-shaped uterus and clear cell adenocarcinoma (CCA) as well as other variations of cerical development. A T-shaped uterus has been associated with a higher risk of ectopic tubal pregnancy and pre-term labor as well as miscarriage.

Men who have been exposed to DES *in utero* have been found to have an increased incidence of epididymal cysts, nondescended testes, hypoplastic testes, varicoceles, and spermatozoal defects. These findings suggest that DES exposure may result in reduced male fertility, but further follow-up studies are needed to determine the extent of any reduction.

After publication of associated concerns between DES and CCA, the FDA issued an alert advising against the use of DES during pregnancy.

Isotretinoin.

Isotretinoin, a vitamin A congener used in the treatment of severe cystic acne, is a potent human teratogen. About 14% of babies born to women who take isotretinoin during the first 10 weeks of pregnancy have cardiac, brain, ear, and other malformations. Isotretinoin also appears to be an abortifacient in humans. The US Food and Drug Administration has estimated that 40% of embryos exposed to isotretinoin during the first trimester are miscarried. As expected, the frequency of miscarriage does not appear to be increased among the pregnancies of women who discontinued isotretinoin therapy prior to conception.

OCCUPATIONAL EXPOSURES AND ENVIRONMENTAL POLLUTANTS

The growing participation of women in the labor force has led to considerable concern about possible hazards to reproduction from exposures in the work place. The unprecedented number of new and increasingly complex chemicals that are polluting the air, water, and food has also given rise to concern about potential reproductive effects of environmental pollutants. Nevertheless, few controlled studies have been conducted to evaluate the effects of such exposures on female fertility or pregnancy maintenance.

Many of the substances that are suspected of lowering a woman's fertility are also thought to affect pregnancy loss. The deleterious reproductive effects of lead have been known for more than a century. Reports from Britain indicated that women working in the pottery and white lead industry during the late nineteenth century were more likely to be sterile or, if they became pregnant, to miscarry than women who were not employed in lead work.

Carbon disulfide exposure among women in the textile industry has been reported to lead to menstrual disorders, decreased fertility, and excess fetal loss. A Finnish study revealed an interesting finding, i.e., textile workers, especially seamstresses who were married to metallurgical workers, had an increased rate of spontaneous miscarriages. The specific exposures that may have contributed to the increased fetal loss were not identified, however.

Women working in rubber, leather, dry cleaning, and other industries where benzene was used as a solvent were historically at risk for chronic benzene poisoning. This condition, although not directly associated with infertility, might interfere with the ability to conceive and maintain a pregnancy, as it is characterized by excessive menstruation, which could lead to severe anemia and hemorrhagic complications during pregnancy.

Toxic waste dumps, such as the Love Canal landfill in New York State, which contains more than 200 organic compounds including dioxin, benzene, and toluene, have also elicited widespread attention. An investigation of adverse pregnancy outcomes among women in the Love Canal area found only a slight increase in spontaneous miscarriages, but the validity of this study has been questioned.

Organic Solvents

Organic solvents are widely used in industry and laboratories. Many organic solvents are readily absorbed via the skin and lungs, so the potential for a high degree of absorption exists in environments that do not adequately protect the worker. An increased risk of miscarriage has been found in some, but not all, studies of female workers in industries in which exposure to organic chemicals is common. The inconsistencies found among these studies make it difficult to draw any firm conclusions and suggest that confounding variables rather than organic chemicals may be responsible for the observed associations.

Paternal Occupational Exposures

Excess heat and exposure to certain chemical and physical agents may lower male fertility. A high scrotal temperature can impede sperm maturation. Suggested causes of elevated scrotal temperature are tight underclothing, frequent hot baths or sauna, and prolonged sitting, as in the case of taxi and truck drivers, but there are limited data to substantiate these associations. The effect of extreme heat on spermatogenesis is thought to be reversible in most cases.

One of the few occupational exposures that have clearly been shown to affect testicular function is dibromochloropropane (DBCP), a soil pesticide. Men employed in the manufacture as well as application of DBCP were found to have depressed sperm counts, with some of the factory workers demonstrating clinical infertility. Whether the sperm count depression is reversible is not clear. Manufacture of DBCP in the United States was discontinued after the toxic effects of this pesticide came to public attention. Ethylene dibromide, which replaced DBCP as a common pesticide, has been under suspicion as well, but to date there is no convincing evidence that it impairs male reproductive potential. Occupational exposure to kepone, as well as unspecified types of pesticides have also been reported to cause impotence and infertility.

Sperm abnormalities and sexual malfunction have been attributed to several other occupational exposures, including lead, chloroprene, carbon disulfide, and synthetic estrogens. Workers in a lead storage battery plant in Rumania were found to have an increased incidence of various spermatozoal defects. It has even been hypothesized that the fall of Rome resulted from sterility in the ruling class caused by excess consumption of lead-contaminated wine. Irradiation can also alter sperm production, but its effect appears to be reversible in many cases. As is the case for women, there are no studies that show that *in utero* irradiation adversely affects subsequent fertility in men.

Paternal exposures have also been linked to spontaneous miscarriages, specifically occupational exposures to anesthetic gases, DBCP, vinyl chloride, dioxin contaminants (Agent Orange), and chloroprene. The available evidence for these effects is limited and conflicting, and further documentation is needed before the role of paternal occupational and environmental exposures in pregnancy loss can be established.

Anesthetic Gases

At least 50,000 women annually undergo anesthesia for surgery in the United States, and some 250,000 people work in medical or dental facilities in which anesthetic gases are used regularly. Very little is known about the effect of anesthetics on miscarriage rates in women who undergo surgery during pregnancy, but an increase in fetal resorption has been observed among pregnant rodents exposed to anesthetic levels of nitrous oxide or a combination of nitrous oxide and halothane.

A weak but significant association between working during pregnancy in jobs in which exposure to anesthetic gases may occur and miscarriage was often observed, but serious methodological weaknesses preclude any firm conclusion regarding the results of these studies. A case-controlled investigation of occupational exposure to volatile anesthetics among nurses who had miscarriages found no significant association.

Mercury

Occupational exposure to mercury is mainly to elemental mercury vapor in plants that manufacture paints, amalgam, and thermometers and to inorganic mercury amalgams in dentistry. Several studies have examined the frequency of miscarriage among workers who are occupationally exposed to mercury, but the results have been inconsistent.

Pesticides

The most publicized suggested association of pesticides with miscarriage concerns the herbicides 2, 4-D and 2, 4, 5-T and their mixture, Agent Orange, which was used extensively by United States military forces in Vietnam. Several epidemiologic studies have now been carried out in populations exposed to these chemicals, and no consistent association with miscarriage has been observed.

NUTRITION AND EXERCISE

Conditions of severe dietary restrictions have been linked with lowered fertility. The birth rate 9 months after the Dutch famine during World War II fell by more than 50 percent, and similar fertility declines have been reported after food crises in seventeenth and eighteenth century Europe as well as in Bangladesh during the mid 1970s. Food deprivation is thought to affect fertility primarily because of the increase in amenorrhea during times of starvation. However, other factors may inhibit fertility during famines, such as psychological stress (see below) and marital separation. Voluntary dietary disturbances, as in the case of anorexia nervosa and bulimia, have also been associated with menstrual disturbances and cessation of menses. There is less of a consensus regarding the effect of moderate chronic malnutrition on fecundity.

In addition to women suffering from severe nutritional deprivation, women athletes, particularly long-distance runners and ballet dancers have been found to experience a high incidence of amenorrhea and anovulatory cycles. Although the menstrual disturbances among the latter groups have been correlated with reduction in weight or body fat, there is also some evidence that physical stress may independently affect circulating levels of reproductive hormones. Because normal menstrual cycles have been found to resume with weight gain and/or cessation of exercise, these generally represent temporary effects on fertility.

Obesity may also be associated with menstrual abnormalities. A retrospective survey in the United States and Canada found that women with prolonged and irregular cycles and reported hirsutism were significantly heavier than those who had regular menstrual cycles and no reported excess growth of facial hair. Furthermore, the occurrence of irregular and prolonged cycles was positively correlated with degree of obesity. In addition, women who had been obese as teenagers were more likely to be nulliparous and have insulin resistance associated with polycystic ovarian disease. Although these findings as well as others suggest that fatty tissue may alter hormonal production, the epidemiologic evidence for an association between obesity and infertility is still limited.

There is also little information about the role of strenuous exercise on fetal loss. A Bulgarian study found no evidence of adverse pregnancy outcomes among its female Olympic athletes, despite the fact that some continued their training and even competition during the first months of pregnancy. Most professional athletes or ballet dancers, however, probably tend to either stop training or restrict their activities once a pregnancy is recognized.

PSYCHOLOGICAL FACTORS

Emotional factors are thought to play a significant role in infertility and pregnancy loss, but lack of rigorous studies precludes quantification of the impact of such factors. Investigation in Sweden found that amenorrheic women reported a higher incidence of stressful life events prior to the onset of amenorrhea than women with normal menstrual cycles. Underlying psychopathology has also been linked to the induction of amenorrhea in the case of patients with anorexia nervosa and perhaps among some patients with galactorrhea-amenorrhea syndrome.

In addition to amenorrhea, emotional stress mediated by the hypothalamic-pituitary-gonadal axis may theoretically result in other ovulatory disorders such as progestational deficiency and irregular ovulation. A study from Belgium suggested that stress might cause infertility through the luteinized unruptured follicle syndrome. Furthermore, lowered fertility may result from sexual disorders, such as vaginismus, and painful intercourse, which may be psychogenic in origin.

In Southern California, studies of patients' moods, optimism and feeling of infertility, social support and self-perceived stress associated with reduced success in Infertility treatment. The live birth rate per egg retrieval was lower as were the number of eggs retrieved and fertilized and embryos transferred. In contrast, a woman's initial optimism about becoming pregnant was associated with an increased number of eggs fertilized and embryos transferred.

Emotional factors have also been linked to pregnancy loss, particularly habitual miscarriage. In a study of habitual aborters and patients whom had no history of spontaneous miscarriage, psychological tests revealed more emotional instability, tension, hostile feelings, and guilt in the former than the latter group. Although psychotherapy has been reported to be successful in treating some habitual aborters, there is no clear evidence that the psychological problems were the underlying cause of the pregnancy losses.

PART III

Treatment—New Hope for Miscarriage Patients

8

Fibroids and Miscarriage

Numerous anatomic abnormalities have been associated with unfavorable pregnancy outcomes. These include uterine fibroids, incompetent cervix, congenital malformations, and uterine synechiae. The diagnosis of abnormal intrauterine anatomy should begin with a Hysterosalpingogram (HSG). This procedure will delineate the contour of the uterine cavity and reveal any filling defects. Ultrasound may also provide a significant contribution for the detection of various conditions that may cause miscarriage. Ultimately, surgery such as Hysteroscopy may be necessary to make an accurate diagnosis, which may explain the source of your miscarriages.

A. FIBROIDS

The incidence of uterine fibroids in the female population is approximately 40%. Fibroids have been implicated in spontaneous miscarriage by studies showing a significant reduction in miscarriage rates following their removal (myomectomy). The incidence of spontaneous miscarriage due to fibroids is not known. The difficulty in diagnosing significant fibroids that impact the uterine cavity make it difficult to assess the number of undiagnosed women who have no other symptoms than infertility or reproductive loss.

Uterine fibroids are usually diagnosed by pelvic examination. A Hysterosalpingogram may reveal filling defects consistent with fibroids within the uterine cavity that cannot be felt by the physician on pelvic examination. Hysteroscopic confirmation may be beneficial both as a diagnostic and therapeutic maneuver because these tumors are often amenable to resection by hysteroscopy.

Uterine fibroids may be associated with repeated pregnancy loss. The mechanisms that cause pain and bleeding with fibroids have been described, but the pathophysiology that results in pregnancy loss may be multiple and yet elusive. Uterine fibroids may be a reason for pregnancy loss, but all other factors that contribute to repeat miscarriage should be excluded prior to surgery. In well-selected patients, myomectomy may improve the prognosis for a normal pregnancy.

What are Fibroids?

Uterine fibroids or fibroids are benign smooth muscle neoplasms that occur in 40% of women over 40 years of age. Fibroids are not common in women under 25 years of age. On the other hand, up to 50% of women have fibroids at the age of 50. Uterine fibroids are therefore prevalent in the late reproductive years. The increasing incidence of these tumors corresponds to an increased risk for spontaneous miscarriage with advanced age.

The incidence of clinically evident spontaneous miscarriages in the general population is estimated to be between 15% and 20%. When pregnancy losses before or at the time of menses are included, 30% to 50% of fertilized ova may be lost. Spontaneous miscarriages may be attributed to genetic abnormalities, hormonal and immunologic causes, medical illness, psychogenic factors, infection, environmental toxins, and uterine factors. With the high incidence of miscarriages and the high prevalence of uterine fibroids, many patients with fibroids may be expected to experience one or more spontaneous miscarriages. Fibroids have been found in 18% of women with two or more miscarriages. When caring for a patient with fibroids and repeated pregnancy loss, a thorough evaluation must be done to identify whether the fibroids may be the cause for miscarriages or unrelated to a patient's poor reproductive history. To understand better the role of fibroids in pregnancy loss, the following serves as insight into the physiology of fibroids, the related functional and mechanical uterine alterations that occur, and the diagnosis and treatment of fibroids.

How Did I Get Fibroids?

Uterine fibroids are derived from smooth muscle tissue. Fibroids tend to be multiple, although each fibroid is believed to be unicellular in origin. Fibroids are responsive to hormones, including estrogen and progesterone, but whether hormones play a role in their origin is uncertain. In women, estrogen stimulates fibroid growth. Estrogen deprivation occurs with menopause or treatment with gonadotropin-releasing hormone analogues (GnRHa) that reduces the fibroid size.

Although estrogen clearly stimulates growth of uterine fibroids, the role of estrogen in the origin of fibroids and the mechanism by which estrogen stimulates fibroid enlargement has not been established with certainty. Progesterone receptors are present in uterine fibroids. Short-term, high-dose progesterone therapy has been shown to cause degeneration of fibroids. Researchers have shown lower doses of progesterone with an antiprogestin RU-486 prior to surgery have associated with fibroid shrinkage.

The effect of physiologic concentrations of progesterone in the stimulation or inhibition of fibroid growth is not clear. Although the high levels of progesterone that occur with pregnancy may cause degeneration in some fibroids, progesterone levels in nonpregnant women are not likely to have a major effect.

Additional endocrine or paracrine hormones may affect growth of fibroids. Growth hormone combined with estrogen causes a synergistic uterine weight gain in rats. Human placental lactogen, which is similar in structure and activity to growth hormone, may accelerate estrogen-induced fibroid growth in pregnancy. Uterine fibroids contain receptors for prostaglandins E and F2alpha and oxytocin. Receptors for epidermal growth factor are present, and epidermal growth factor may stimulate fibroid growth. Despite the demonstration of receptors for these factors in fibroids, a direct role has not been established to explain the role of these substances in the origin of fibroids or symptoms produced by these tumors.

How Do Fibroids Cause Miscarriage?

Uterine fibroids may cause pregnancy loss by one or more mechanisms. Mechanical factors may contribute to pregnancy loss depending on tumor size and location. Fibroids may alter the vascular supply to the implanting embryo or growing pregnancy. The vascular supply may be progressively compromised by fibroid growth during pregnancy. Uterine fibroids may also alter the endometrium. Uterine irritability due to fibroids may interfere with embryo implantation; result in early miscarriage or cause premature labor.

How Important are the Location of Fibroids?

The location of uterine fibroids is the most important factor to consider for patients with spontaneous miscarriage. Fibroids may be found in three locations: submucosal (inner uterine cavity), intramural (in the wall of uterus) or subserosal (outer uterine wall). Subserosal and intramural fibroids that cause no distortion of the uterine cavity are less likely to cause miscarriage in contrast to submucosal or intramural fibroids that distort the uterus. Uterine cavity distortion is present in 56% of the hysterectomy specimens in infertility patients and in 22% on hysterosalpingogram (HSG). Fibroids that distort the uterine cavity may directly interfere with implantation and cause expulsion of the fertilized ovum. Submucosal fibroids or intramural fibroids may alter the endometrium and inhibit implantation. Vascular supply to the implantation site may be affected by fibroids that distort the uterine cavity.

The location of fibroids is important as pregnancy progresses. Bleeding in early pregnancy, premature rupture of membranes, and postpartum hemorrhage are more likely to occur when the placenta is implanted near a fibroid. Fibroids located in the lower uterine segment are associated with a higher frequency of cesarean section and retained placenta. Fibroids under the placenta may predispose to displacement of the placenta with bleeding and possible separation of the placenta (placental abruption).

Example of Subserosal, Intramural and Submucosal Fibroids

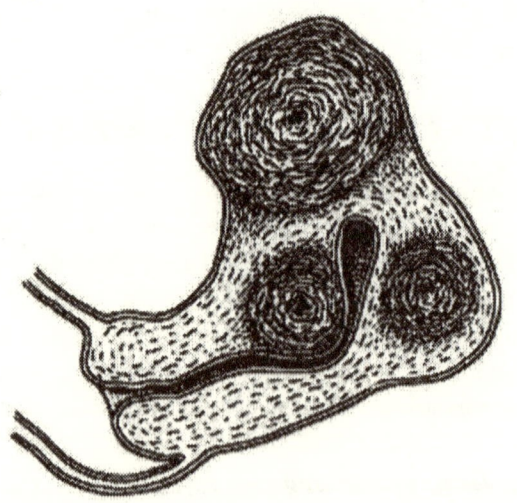

How Important is Fibroid Size?

Fibroids greater than 5 cm especially those that compress the uterine cavity, may be associated with infertility, miscarriage, bleeding in pregnancy, premature labor, premature rupture of membranes, pain, and postpartum bleeding.

The consideration of the combined effects of size and location of fibroids is important for patients with recurrent pregnancy loss. Small submucosal fibroids are more likely to be an important cause of pregnancy loss than a large tumor that does not physically compromise the uterine cavity. Large intramural or submucosal fibroids that result in significant endometrial distortion warrant treatment in patients with recurrent pregnancy loss.

Alterations in the endometrium may be a cause of fetal loss due to fibroids. A number of endometrial abnormalities have been found with fibroids. Pressure atrophy, usually but not always at the endometrium overlying the fibroid, was found in one fourth of the specimens. Ulceration of the endometrium was noted in less than 10% of the specimens.

A much higher incidence of topographic endometrial abnormalities are found with submucosal fibroids. Total endometrial glandular atrophy has been identified in the endometrium overlying submucosal fibroids as well as the area directly opposite a submucosal fibroid. The endometrium remote from the submucosal fibroid had a lower incidence of atrophy but a high percentage of histologic abnormalities. Although the mucosa over submucosal fibroids demonstrate the most dramatic changes of glandular atrophy and thinning, tumors at other sites cause endometrial changes. Intramural fibroids may cause marked thickening and hypertrophy of the endometrium, especially in the depressions between tumor nodules. Fibroids that cause endometrial atrophy may provide a poor implantation site for the blastocyst embryo and result in early pregnancy loss. Subtle endometrial alterations may increase the risk of miscarriage, although cause-and-effect relationships are difficult to prove.

Alterations in uterine blood flow may cause pregnancy loss in some women with fibroids. The relationship of fibroids to abnormal endometrial veins has clarified the venous dilatation and congestion that results from compression of venous plexus in myometrium and endometrium adjacent to fibroids. Size and location are important considerations with large submucosal fibroids that produce the most striking venous congestion, whereas small subserosal tumors may have no effect. Endometrial and myometrial venous congestion may alter the endometrial environment in such a way as to prevent implantation of the fertilized egg and result in infertility or pregnancy loss.

Studies of regional blood flow in fibroids reveals a lower blood flow in fibroids than in myometrium of the same uterus. It seems reasonable that a decreased blood supply to the developing placenta may ultimately contribute to spontaneous miscarriage. In addition, growth of a fibroid or surrounding tissue during a pregnancy may compromise blood flow to a fibroid. Degeneration of the fibroid and uterine irritability may result from inadequate circulation and predispose to pregnancy loss.

Uterine irritability as a result of fibroids may increase the risk of miscarriage. Submucosal or intramural fibroids larger than 2 cm may irritate the uterus, increase uterine contractility, and cause separation and expulsion of an early pregnancy.

What Other Symptoms May I Have With Fibroids?

Most patients with fibroids are asymptomatic, even in pregnancy. Common symptoms associated with fibroids are heavier periods, longer periods, pelvic pain, pelvic pressure, pain with intercourse, and urinary urgency or frequency. Patients with fibroids may experience infertility. Abdominal bloating and constipation may occur as a result of bowel compression. Fatigue caused by anemia due to heavy bleeding may occur.

How Can I Find Out if I Have Uterine Fibroids?

Fibroids should be considered for all patients who experience pregnancy loss. Traditionally, diagnosis has relied on a history and physical examination. Overall, only 38% of fibroids are detected by pelvic examination at the time of the initial obstetrical visit. Approximately one fourth of fibroids less than 5 cm are palpated, and just over half of the tumors over 5 cm are detected. Small or centrally located fibroids may escape detection in the uterus. Pelvic examination, although very helpful, is by no means foolproof in diagnosing fibroid tumors. Moreover, in patients with fibroids, it is usually impossible to determine if the tumors present are located in or near the uterine cavity. Further diagnostic studies are necessary.

Hysterosalpingogram (HSG) is advised for all patients with recurrent pregnancy loss. The HSG provides considerable information regarding location, size, and number of submucosal and intramural fibroids Submucosal and intramural fibroids often cause enlargement of the uterine cavity. Fibroids may distort the normal triangular shape of the cavity and may manifest as filling defects in the uterus. Fibroids may cause obstruction of the fallopian tubes, and submucous tumors are among the causes of heavier menses.

A HSG or hysteroscopy should be performed in the nongravid state when the suspicion of a uterine fibroid has been raised. The HSG cannot show the precise size or location of the fibroid. Hysteroscopy provides a more exact impression of the characteristics of the tumor. Abnormalities found on hysterosalpingography may not always be confirmed by hysteroscopy. Laparoscopy in combination with hysteroscopy provides the most thorough evaluation of the uterus in patients with suspected fibroids and recurrent pregnancy loss.

Ultrasound, computed tomography (CT) scan, and magnetic resonance imaging (MRI) have greatly increased the ability to diagnose and localize fibroids. Laparoscopy and hysteroscopy may provide direct visualization as minor surgical procedures.

Sonography is widely used to diagnose or to confirm the diagnosis of fibroids. In the nonpregnant patient, the most common abnormalities are contour irregularity, altered echo density, and uterine enlargement. Twenty percent to 40% of patients with fibroids have no sonographic abnormalities, although most patients with fibroids larger than 2 cm have sonographic abnormalities. A condition known as Adenomyosis may have a similar impact as fibroids, yet be difficult to diagnosis by diagnostic tests. A sonohysterogram (SHG) may be performed to improve the accuracy of submucosal fibroid detection with the uterine cavity. During this procedure, sterile saline in placed into the uterine cavity while performing an ultrasound that improves the physician's ability to evaluate the walls of the uterus.

Advanced imaging techniques such as MRI and CT have been used to evaluate the change in fibroid size with therapy. Magnetic resonance imaging is preferable to CT for pelvic imaging because the former provides no interference from pelvic bones, allows the ability to reconstruct images in several planes, and provides the ability to change soft-tissue contrast. This allows MRI to demonstrate fibroids in relation to the uterine cavity with more detail than is possible with CT scanning or ultrasound. Magnetic resonance imaging offers the disadvantages of being time-consuming and expensive, and it fails to provide the clinically relevant detail of HSG or hysteroscopy. Magnetic resonance imaging remains a valuable tool, but its place in the routine clinical evaluation for fibroids is not yet established.

How Should Fibroids be Treated?

A woman with recurrent pregnancy loss or infertility should have a comprehensive evaluation. Other causative factors should be addressed prior to or in conjunction with the treatment of fibroids. Although it is difficult to prove that fibroids are the cause of early pregnancy loss, therapy for fibroids may be warranted in a woman with repeated pregnancy loss in whom all other factors have been eliminated by a thorough investigation. Only after all other factors have been eliminated should surgery be considered for the enhancement of pregnancy outcome in a woman with fibroids. Surgery remains the definitive therapy of choice for fibroids in a woman wishing to maximize her fertility.

Hysteroscopic resection of submucosal fibroids may be performed with excellent results. A resectoscope utilized with a fluid-distending medium is usually employed with Laparoscopy to avoid uterine perforation

To perform hysteroscopic myomectomy, the location of the tumor should first be confirmed. A preoperative Ultrasound or HSG helps demonstrate the relationship of the fibroid to the uterotubal Os and lower uterine segment. The resectoscope is used to shave down the tumor to its base.

Hysteroscopic resection allows for the removal of submucosal fibroids and removal of sessile tumors to the level of the endometrial lining. Uterine perforation, infection, and cautery injury are risks of hysteroscopic surgery. Morbidity has been low for this procedure compared to abdominal myomectomy, however.

Why Might My Doctor Advise an Abdominal Myomectomy?

Abdominal myomectomy is indicated in women with symptomatic fibroids who desire uterine preservation. Women with recurrent pregnancy loss may benefit from an abdominal myomectomy when the fibroids cause significant distortion of the uterine cavity as demonstrated by hysteroscopy or HSG. All women should complete a thorough evaluation to determine other possible causes of infertility and pregnancy loss before a myomectomy is performed.

The operative technique of myomectomy is based on the observation that fibroids displace myometrium as they enlarge. This displacement results in a distortion of the uterus rather than invasion of the myometrium.

The uterine incision is made so that as many fibroids as possible may be removed through a single incision. A single anterior vertical incision is the most useful in exposing as many fibroids as possible while posing the lowest likelihood of adhesion formation. Many inaccessible tumors can be removed through this incision by pushing the fibroid toward the incision and removing it through this central incision. Occasionally, however, two or three incisions may be required for complete removal of multiple fibroid tumors.

Various methods have been described to reduce blood loss during a uterine myomectomy. Vasopressin may be injected directly into the myometrium around the base of fibroids to minimize blood loss. Vasopressin reduces the need for blood transfusion during myomectomy, but it does not mask arterial bleeding. Careful dissection, prompt suturing, and the use of direct pressure to bleeding vessels aid in minimizing blood loss. Antilogous blood may be made available for patients undergoing myomectomy.

How May A Surgeon Reduce Scar Tissue Formation After a Myomectomy?

Additional techniques have been advocated to minimize postoperative adhesion formation. Interceed (Johnson & Johnson, New Brunswick, NJ), an absorbable adhesion barrier, has been shown to reduce adhesion formation on the pelvic sidewall. Its efficacy for uterine defects is not known, but the barrier must not be used unless complete homeostasis has been established. Gore-Tex (WL Gore & Associates, Inc, Flagstaff, AZ) surgical membrane can be sutured directly over the uterine serial incision after homeostasis has been established. A "second-look" laparoscopy with adhesiolysis may also be useful to reduce adhesions when performed soon after the initial procedure.

What Improvement Can I Expect After A Myomectomy?

Spontaneous miscarriage rates reduce from 41% preoperatively to 19% after myomectomy, a figure that approaches the rate of pregnancy loss in the general population. The term pregnancy rate following myomectomy for repeated pregnancy loss approaches 50%. This rate is comparable to the 30% to 50% term pregnancy rate expected after myomectomy in women with primary infertility. Significant improvements in pregnancy rates after abdominal myomectomy for patients with a submucosal fibroid greater than 5 cm are seen.

Can I Still Have a Vaginal Delivery After a Myomectomy?

Many gynecologists advocate cesarean section following extensive myomectomy or entry into the uterine cavity. Potential weakening of the uterine wall may lead to silent separation of the original incision area at the time of labor jeopardizing the health of the baby if vaginal delivery is attempted.

What is the Role of a GnRH Analogue?

The role of GnRH analogues in the management of uterine fibroids is controversial. Gonadotropin-releasing hormone analogue therapy resulted in significant reduction of uterine volume. By 6 months after therapy, all volumes return to baseline levels. Side effects of GnRH analogue therapy commonly experienced are hot flashes, decreased breast size, vaginal dryness, fatigue, and insomnia. Less common symptoms include decreased libido, depression, irregular bleeding, local reaction, and weight gain. Bone density decreases during therapy, but this effect is partially or completely reversible after treatment is discontinued. Although symptomatic improvement often persists in women after GnRH analogue therapy of fibroids despite uterine re-enlargement, a direct therapeutic benefit in women with habitual miscarriage is doubtful. Rather, GnRH analogue therapy may be useful for anemic women with fibroids to restore hemoglobin to normal levels prior to surgery. Shrinkage of large submucous fibroids with GnRH analogues may allow for easier hysteroscopic removal or may facilitate abdominal myomectomy.

CONCLUSION

Fibroids may be the occasional cause of repeat pregnancy loss or subfertility, especially when the tumors are large and cause significant alteration of the uterine cavity. The mechanism of pregnancy loss may involve changes in blood flow; placental abruption is also common with submucous fibroids. The development of new surgical techniques such as hysteroscopic resection of submucosal fibroids and preoperative GnRH analogue therapy may greatly reduce surgical morbidity. Hysteroscopic myomectomy is advocated to remove pedunculated and small submucous fibroids. Myomectomy is usually advisable for women with recurrent miscarriages when a thorough investigation has eliminated all other factors. Uterine fibroids are usually asymptomatic during pregnancy, but circumstantial evidence suggests an association with threatened miscarriage and preterm labor if left untreated.

9

Anatomy—Ways to Correct Pregnancy Loss

Uterine Causes of Miscarriage

A. UTERINE MALFORMATIONS

Uterine or "Mullerian duct" malformations constitute an interesting and challenging group of clinical problems for the obstetrician-gynecologist. In most patients, uterine anomalies are asymptomatic and remain undetected, whereas in others, the untoward consequence of repetitive pregnancy loss yields evidence of their presence. It is in the area of pregnancy loss that uterine anomalies have generated the most attention. Fetal loss is increased in all trimesters. Midtrimester miscarriage of a normal fetus, premature labor, and abnormal fetal presentation are conditions classically associated with breech presentation which is increased from 3.7% in women without a uterine anomaly to 20% women who do exhibit one. Abdominal delivery and postpartum complications, including retained placenta and hemorrhage, are also more frequent.

How Would I Know If I Have a Uterine Malformation?

Approximately 75% of all reproductive losses precede clinical awareness. A concerning obstetric history is accepted as an indication to search for uterine malformations. Establishing the diagnosis of a congenital uterine anomaly as the cause of pregnancy loss follows a systematic approach.

Table 1. Gynecologic and Obstetric History and Findings of Uterine Anomalies

<u>Gynecologic consideration of uterine anomaly in women with the following:</u>

- Oligoamenonhea with persistent dysmenorrhea

- Chronic pelvic pain

- Persistent dysfunctional uterine bleeding

- Persistent painful sex

- History of infertility

- Recurrent urinary tract infections

- In utero exposure to diethylstilbestrol

<u>Obstetric consideration of mullerian anomaly in women with the following:</u>

- History of repetitive pregnancy loss

- History of poor obstetric outcome

- Ectopic pregnancy

- Premature labor

- Abnormal presentation in labor

- Intrapartum complications at delivery

- Postpartum hemorrhage

- Retained placenta

- Incompetent cervix

- Previous infant with intrauterine growth retardation

<u>Findings on Pelvic Examinations:</u>

- Presence of widened fundus on bimanual

- Symptomatic or asymptomatic pelvic mass

- Vaginal or cervical abnormality

Mullerian Anomalies

The mullerian or paramesonephric ducts, which are evident by the end of the second month of gestation, ultimately fuse to form the uterus, cervix, and upper four fifths of the vagina. Incomplete fusion of these ducts results in uterine anomalies that may be associated with recurrent pregnancy loss. Examples include unicornuate, bicornuate, didelphic, and septate uteri

The incidence of mullerian abnormalities in the general population is difficult to assess because asymptomatic women do not routinely present for evaluation. The best estimates, ranging from 1.9% to 6.2%, have been derived from studies in which pelvic or abdominal procedures have been carried out for other indications. Mullerian abnormalities have been implicated in fetal loss in approximately 10% of couples that present for evaluation of their reproductive failure. The most common anomalies are unicornuate, bicornuate, and septate uteri. The greatest incidence of fetal loss has been demonstrated in association with the septate uterus, with estimates as high as 67% to 85%. The increased rate of fetal loss may be related to insufficient endometrial blood flow. The incidence of miscarriage in selected patients with bicornuate and unicornuate uteri ranges from 21% to 41%. Reduced cavity size is thought to contribute to pregnancy loss in all these abnormalities. The risk of fetal loss in patients with arcuate uteri is probably no higher than that of the general population; this "anomaly" is felt to represent a normal variant of uterine architecture.

The treatment of mullerian anomalies is surgical. A uterine septum is best treated via hysteroscopic resection. This method involves incision of the fibromuscular septum under direct visualization using hysteroscopic scissors or a resectoscope. Other procedures, now less frequently used, include the Tompkins metroplasty and the Jones metroplasty. In the Jones metroplasty, the uterine septum is excised as a wedge in the anteroposterior plane and repaired in the same manner as the Strassman procedure. The Tompkins metroplasty involves a single median incision through the septum to the level of the endometrial cavity with reapproximation of the myometrium anteriorly and posteriorly. The bicornuate uterus, in the setting of recurrent miscarriage with an otherwise negative work-up, is best treated by the Strassman procedure. This involves incising the two uterine fundi in a transverse fashion to the level of the endometrium. The myometrial edges are then reapproximated at right angles to the initial incision to create a unified endometrial cavity. Many authors discourage repair of the didelphic uterus owing to technical difficulties and poor outcome.

1) Septate Uterus

Septate uterus is generally associated with poor obstetric outcome. Diminished blood supply, distortion of the cavity, and associated cervical hormonal abnormalities may all be responsible for increased pregnancy loss. Abdominal metroplasty is not recommended owing to the heightened risk of postoperative adhesions, infertility, and need for cesarean section. Hysteroscopic resection of the septum is a safe and effective alternative.

The most impressive feature of a septate uterus is the pregnancy loss noted in the first half of pregnancy. In the series of Buttram and Gibbons, 88% of pregnancy associated with complete septum ended in miscarriage, as did 70% associated with the incomplete form. It is possible that the more complete the septum, the greater the probability of miscarriage.

Figure 1

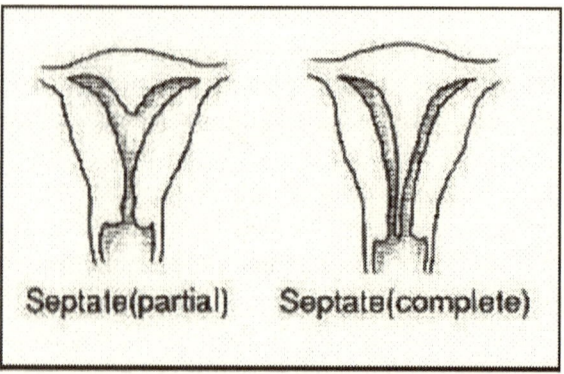

Septate(partial)   Septate(complete)

With the septate uterus, which is the most common anomaly associated with fetal loss, fetal loss typically declines from 88% to 12% following therapy. Prior to unification of surgical therapy, a complete infertility evaluation should be performed to identify any other infertility factors such as obstruction of the fallopian tubes, luteal phase defects, anovulation, poor sperm quality, and so forth.

2) Double Uterus

The bicornuate or double uterus is associated with a 20% incidence of premature labor, breech presentation, and cesarean section. Premature labor is a particular problem in this group who deliver on the average at 35 weeks. The incidence of miscarriage is increased, but an exact figure is difficult to obtain because many reported series failed to separate the patients with bicornuate uteri from those with a septate uterus. In series reporting fetal loss rates for bicornuate uteri, the rates vary from 40% to 90%. The recommended therapy for a double uterus associated with repeat reproductive loss is the Strassman procedure, which has the advantage of not requiring excision of uterine tissue and, thus, not reducing the potential volume of the uterine cavity.

Figure 2

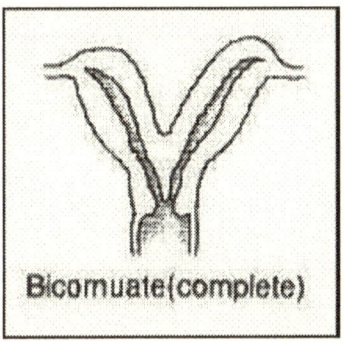

Bicornuate(complete)

3) Unicornuate Uterus

There is an increased incidence of abnormal mullerian duct development in women who have recurrent miscarriages. Unicornuate uterus is one such defect. Routine prophylactic cervical cerclage in unicornuate uterine pregnancies is controversial. Pregnancy outcome is better in uterus didelphys than in unicornuate uterus owing to the better blood supply through collateral connection between the two horns. Patients with a bicornuate uterus have a 60% likelihood of a successful pregnancy outcome, but they are at high risk of cervical incompetence. Cervical cerclage is not recommended routinely for these patients, but should be placed if the cervix is found to be shortened or dilated on transvaginal ultrasound during pregnancy.

Renal imaging via intravenous pyelography (IVP) or ultrasonography should be considered for women with a unicornuate uterus. The reported rate of renal anomalies approaches 66%, with the most common being absence of one kidney.

Figure 3

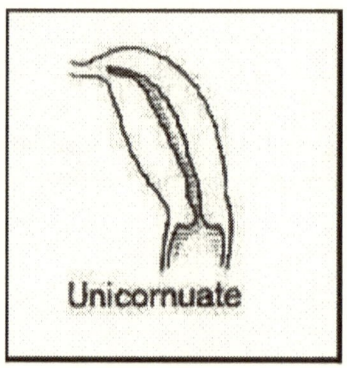

How Do These Uterine Changes Occur?

Simply stated, mullerian anomalies represent a group of congenital uterine mal-formations that result from abnormal formation, arrested development, or incomplete fusion of the uterine ducts. From a more anatomic and physiologic point of view, the defects result from failure of initial descent, fusion, and resorp-tion of the uterine septum.

How Do Women With These Changes Miscarry?

The association between the presence of a uterine anomaly and pregnancy loss is well known, and estimates of approximately 15 to 20% are in the medical litera-ture. Inadequate uterine volume for the products of conception with increased pressure on the lower uterine segment and cervix is believed to play a role in pre-mature pregnancy losses. Much emphasis has been placed on the poor prognosis of implantation of the septum. The reduced vascularity the septum is felt to be inadequate for proper placental perfusion and pregnancy maintenance; thereby leading to early pregnancy was age. A third theory implicates increased uterine irritability and contractility associated with alterations in serum cystine ami-nopeptides that lead to premature cervical thinning and dilatation or conse-quences of placental insufficiency that lead to pregnancy loss is theorized that the more complete the uterine septum, the higher the incidence of first-trimester miscarriage.

How Can An Accurate Diagnosis Be Made?

With the rapid expansion in reproductive technologies, an increased awareness of the many uses of ultrasound in pelvic conditions has followed. Although most clinicians still rely on hysterosalpingography to establish the presence or absence of a particular uterine abnormality, others are looking into the applicability of ultrasonographic techniques for easier, more comfortable, and less expensive means of establishing a diagnosis of mullerian abnormality. The role of MRI imaging with regard to the diagnosis of mullerian anomalies may provide significant help when findings on physical examination, hysterosalpinography, and ultrasonography remain equivocal. Ultimately, an accurate diagnosis (and therapy) may require the performance of a laparoscopy and hysteroscopy.

What is a DES Uterus?

Intrauterine changes were observed women with known in utero exposure to Diethylstilbestrol (DES). Ninety percent of patients who had DES cervical changes had hysterosalpingogram abnormalities. Eighteen percent of those who had a normal-appearing cervix had changes on hysterosalpingogram. The clinical importance of these findings relates to early studies demonstrating an increased incidence of premature labor. Women with DES exposure may benefit from a cervical cerclage if thinning of the cervix is observed.

Treatment of pregnancy loss associated with several of the classes of anomalies with cervical cerclage alone, with fetal salvage rates comparable to the more complicated surgical procedures. Certainly, in those malformations associated with a functional hemiuterus, such as a didelphus or unicornuate uterus, this can be very useful. It is possible that more widespread experience with this therapy may change therapy recommendations in the future.

SUMMARY

Although not common, mullerian malformations are one of the more successfully treatable forms of pregnancy loss. For this reason, this particular form of gynecologic abnormality remains a challenge. With the continued improvements in medical technology of the past decade, newer diagnostic capabilities have allowed clinicians a closer investigative view at etiologies causing repetitive pregnancy loss. In addition, potential management options have progressed to a more conservative, less expensive, and safer outpatient care for patients, yielding results that are equally as effective as those achieved with major operative procedures of the past. A heightened degree of clinical suspicion, coupled with an increased use of advanced reproductive medicine technologies as hysterosalpingograms, pelvic ultrasounds, and hysteroscopic and laparoscopic techniques, will able the clinician to diagnose these uterine abnormalities. Successful treatment options are available for many of the mullerian anomalies, and there is currently a trend toward more conservative approaches.

B. ASHERMAN'S SYNDROME

My Doctor Told Me I Have Scar Tissue In My Uterus—What is This Syndrome?

Intrauterine synechiae (Asherman's syndrome) are adhesions within the uterine cavity, causing partial or complete obliteration of the cavity. The approximate incidence of intrauterine adhesions in the general population is 2%. This condition usually occurs as a result of prior uterine instrumentation or infection. The most frequently cited predisposing factor is prior uterine curettage, especially following pregnancy. Twenty-two percent of cases were associated with postpartum curettage, with the majority following term pregnancy in patients who had undergone curettage during the second to fourth week postpartum. Pelvic infection has also been associated with synechiae.

Asherman's syndrome is an acquired uterine disorder characterized by uterine adhesions leading to menstrual disorders, infertility, and possibly pregnancy loss. Miscarriage may be due to impaired implantation secondary to intrauterine fibrosis and endometrial inflammation. Up to 88% of patients with Asherman's syndrome have undergone postabortal or postpartum uterine curettage. Amenorrhea or hypomenorrhea are present in 75% of women with this condition. Hysterosalpingography is indicated in suspected cases, but definitive diagnosis requires hysteroscopy. Hysteroscopically directed adhesiolysis is the preferred surgical treatment.

The common denominator appears to be denudation and subsequent fibrosis of the basalis layer, almost always between 1 to 3 weeks postpartum or postmiscarriage; endometrial regeneration fails to occur normally, and uterine adhesions result. Nongestational trauma, surgery (myomectomy, dilatation and curettage, intrauterine device insertion), or specific infections (genital tuberculosis, endometritis) account for far fewer cases. Although the softer, gravid uterus is more vulnerable to curettage-induced denudation of the basalis layer, the increased incidence of IUA following missed miscarriages may be due to the stimulation of fibroblastic activity by retained placental tissue, favoring endometrial fibrosis over regeneration.

How Can Asherman's Syndrome be Diagnosed?

Intrauterine adhesions may cause repeat miscarriage. The diagnosis of intrauterine adhesions, which should be suspected in women with very light menstrual periods, is made by demonstrating the characteristic intrauterine filling defects on hysterosalpingogram.

Direct visualization afforded by hysteroscopy makes it a more reliable and efficient diagnostic tool for differentiating intrauterine adhesions (IUA) from other filling defects that may be present within the endometrial cavity. This contrasts with the Hysterosalpingogram (HSG) x-ray, which may be plagued with inaccuracy or misinterpretation. Most recently, a comprehensive classification scheme integrating HSG and endoscopy findings has been proposed by the Society of Reproductive Surgeons and may provide important uniformity and consistency to the reporting and classification of IUA.

How Is Asherman's Syndrome Treated?

Probably the most widely used protocol today involves hysteroscopic lysis of adhesions. One month of postoperative steroids (Premarin, 1.25-2.5 mg daily for days 1-21, with supplemental medroxyprogesterone acetate on days 16-21) is presumed to enhance endometrial regeneration. Attempts at conception are encouraged following a post-operative HSG to document improvement.

Asherman's syndrome has also been shown to be treated effectively by simple dilatation and curettage. Regardless of the approach utilized, hysteroscopic inspection of the cavity at the conclusion of the procedure should be performed to document adequacy of treatment. Most authorities advocate temporary placement of an intrauterine IUD or foley to minimize postoperative adherence of the uterine walls during healing. Often, a brief course of postoperative estrogen is given to enhance re-epithelialization of the endometrium.

Adhesiolysis with the operative hysteroscope, under laparoscopic guidance and in conjunction with postoperative estrogen, has become the protocol of choice for lysing and preventing reformation of intrauterine adhesions. Operating time is short (approximately 30 to 45 minutes), complications extremely rare (bleeding, infection rates <1%), and results excellent, with restoration of menses in over 90% of patients and an overall pregnancy rate of 79%, with fetal viability achieved in 96%.

What Other Symptom's Occur in Asherman's Syndrome?

The most common symptom is sterility, present in approximately 43% of patients with documented disease. Less common sequelae include early habitual miscarriage (14%), whereas other pregnancy-related complications, such as placenta acreta, previa, or preterm labor and delivery, represent a significant proportion of deliveries during the third trimester. Menstrual abnormalities may range from amenorrhea (37%) or hypomenorrhea (31%), to dysmenorrhea or menometrorrhagia (<5%), or, in fact, menses may be entirely normal. Again, however, because the incidence of IUA is unknown in asymptomatic, fertile women, we must be cautious when assigning cause-and-effect relationships, particularly in the setting of infertility or pregnancy loss.

A Case example

A 38-year-old woman who had undergone a dilatation and curettage for retained placental products 2 weeks following an uneventful vaginal delivery and subsequently experienced a first-and second-trimester spontaneous miscarriage.

Hysteroscopy is a useful adjunct to a hysterosalpingogram (HSG) in the diagnosis of Asherman's syndrome. Only a fair correlation exists between hysterograms and hysteroscopic findings. Therefore uterine abnormalities suggested on hysterogram should be confirmed by direct hysteroscopic visualization.

Hysteroscopy is used not only as an important diagnostic tool but also as a therapeutic measure in the event that intrauterine adhesions are found. Hysteroscopic resection of the scar tissue is performed under anesthesia. Several studies have demonstrated that hysteroscopic lysis of intrauterine adhesions improves subsequent pregnancy outcome.

C. CERVICAL INCOMPETENCE

The cervix is said to be incompetent when it is unable to maintain a pregnancy to term. Its incidence among habitual aborters is variously reported from 8% to 15%.

What is an Incompetent Cervix?

The classic history of cervical incompetence is one of repetitive, acute, painless, second-trimester pregnancy loss without associated bleeding or contractions. This usually presents with spontaneous rupture of the membranes or bulging of the membranes into the vagina. Although some patients present with the classic silent dilatation, others may experience urinary frequency, lower abdominal pressure, a bearing-down sensation, bloody show, or a profuse, watery discharge.

Attempts at diagnosis in the nonpregnant state have included passage of a no.8 Hegar dilator, measurement of resistance through the internal Os with traction on an inflated Foley catheter, hysterosalpingography, and measurement of the minimal electrical current needed to stimulate muscular contraction. In general, these methods have not gained wide clinical acceptance. Furthermore, because attempts to correct cervical incompetence prior to conception have been shown to decrease fertility rates by almost 50%, so the need for diagnosis in the non-pregnant state may be seriously questioned.

When a pregnant patient presents with the classic history just described, few would argue the decision to proceed with a prophylactic cerclage. However, when the primigravida thought to be at high-risk presents, or a patient's history of prior pregnancy loss does not exactly fit the classic description for cervical incompetence, the decision to proceed with therapy is less clear. The presence of a dilated cervix on physical examination does not universally imply cervical incompetence or impending preterm labor. Both serial cervical examinations and serial ultrasound studies have been advocated in this setting.

My Doctor States I Should Have a Cerclage Placed. What Types of Techniques May Be Performed?

The list of therapies proposed for the patient with recurrent pregnancy loss due to cervical incompetence is lengthy and diverse, Included are such techniques as electrocautery of the internal us, scarification with benzoin and talc, obliteration of the endocervical glands with a motorized wire brush followed by complete surgical closure of the cervix as well as various hormones, pessaries, and intravaginal balloons, however, the mainstay of current therapy is surgical cerclage. Even so, the list of procedures remains long, with over 35 different cerclage techniques published to date. Although each differs in some manner, most are variations on one of three major procedures: the Shirodkar, McDonald, or transabdominal cervicoisthmic cerclage.

Shirodkar Technique

Since Shirodkar first introduced his operation in 1955. The suture material is synthetic woven surgical tape with attached atraumatic needles. In general, after 37 weeks' gestation, the cerclage is cut and either removed or left in situ to work itself out during labor.

McDonald Cerclage

The suture should be large and nonabsorbable, such as the Mersilene tape mentioned previously. The cerclage should be placed well posteriorly, as close to the uterosacral ligaments as possible without traversing the cul de sac. Each bite is placed deep enough to include cervical connective tissue with care taken not to enter the endocervical canal. The knot is usually placed anteriorly, with the two free ends left long enough to allow easy removal later in pregnancy.

Transabdominal Cervicoisthmic Cerclage

Transabdominal cervicoisthmic cerclage was first advocated in 1965 for patients who were deemed poor candidates for a vaginal procedure. Such patients as those with (1) an obvious congenitally short or extensively amputated cervix; (2) marked scarring of the cervix or (3) deeply notched multiple cervical defects. Similar to most other therapies for cervical incompetence, the success rate when compared to each patient's prior obstetric history seems impressive. Summarizing all of the published series to date, Marx noted an improvement in salvage rate from 16% to 85% with the use of transabdominal cerclage. No prospective or randomized series of this procedure have been published.

The procedure involves a Pfannenstiel incision (like that for most cesarean sections), and Mersilene tape is then passed around the lower uterine segment.

Although this may be the procedure of choice in a select few patients with cervical incompetence, several disadvantages are readily apparent. Not only is laparotomy required for placement, but a second laparotomy and is required for delivery because the band cannot usually be removed vaginally. Furthermore, should a miscarriage or intrauterine demise occur, a laparotomy is still needed to deliver the baby. Other disadvantages include the risk of hemorrhage from the dilated parametrial vessels during dissection, potential compromise of uterine vascular supply, and a procedure-related fetal loss rate.

For What Reasons Should A Cerclage Not Be Placed?

Contraindications to cervical cerclage include active bleeding, preterm labor, ruptured membranes, chorioamnionitis, polyhydramnios, and lethal fetal amnionitis. Most workers agree that, beyond 26 weeks' gestation, cerclage should not be offered because neonatal survival at this age is now substantially better than 50%.

Some have suggested that cerclage is also contraindicated when the patient presents with a widely dilated cervix. Several authors have reported success rates less than 50% when a cerclage is performed in this setting. Unfortunately, once the cervix is markedly dilated and the membranes are hourglassed into the vagina, the prognosis without treatment is universally poor.

Pregnancy Outcome with Cervical Cerclage

Most reports that claim to show an improvement in pregnancy outcome with cerclage have done so by comparing salvage rates before and after the procedure using each patient as her own historical control. Tabulating all 61 such series published to date, reported improvement in pregnancy success rates from 21% to 76% with the Shirodkar procedure, from 23% to 74% with McDonald's cerclage, and from 24% to 86% with transabdominal cervicoisthmic cerclage. Interestingly, when reported in this manner, all therapies, whether hormonal, mechanical, or surgical, are associated with success rates of 75% to 90%. Additionally, the chances of a successful pregnancy outcome in patients with two or more consecutive losses can be as high as 79% with no therapy at all.

Summary

Although rare in the general population, cervical incompetence makes up 8% to 15% of women with chronic pregnancy loss. Factors predisposing to cervical incompetence include in utero DES exposure, extensive conization of the cervix, obstetric trauma, and possibly rapid, excessive dilation of the internal Os for elective miscarriage. Although many schemes for diagnosing or predicting the disorder have been proposed, the gold standard remains a classic history of repetitive, painless, midtrimester pregnancy loss. Treatment of the patient with an incompetent cervix is primarily surgical, and no one procedure is demonstrably superior to another. Preoperative antibiotics and tocolytic agents may be used to augment therapeutic or emergent cerclage, but they are not necessary for prophylactic procedures. Complications of cerclage include preterm rupture of the membranes, premature labor, an increased need for hospitalization, and an increased risk of infectious morbidity for both the mother and the neonate. Review of the few randomized controlled trials of cervical cerclage reported to date fails to disclose a clinically significant improvement in preterm birth or neonatal mortality. Consequently, in view of the procedure-related morbidity, there is a clear need for properly designed, randomized, clinical trials to study patients at high risk for cervical incompetence.

10

Infection and Pregnancy Loss

In order to affirmatively establish a cause-and-effect relationship between a particular organism and recurrent miscarriage, as a minimum, infection must be documented in the mother, the placenta, and the fetal tissues. However, few studies exist in the literature that detail pathologic findings to this extent. In addition, the desired epidemiologic studies of association and the treatment studies documenting improved outcome are sparse. Current and historic literature on Mycoplasma, toxoplasmosis, Listeria, Chlamydia, and group B streptococcus is reviewed. These organisms are associated with perinatal infections or adverse outcomes with varying prevalence.

MYCOPLASMAS

Twelve of 64 classified mycoplasmas have been isolated from the respiratory and genitourinary tracts of humans. *Mycoplasma hominis* and *Ureaplasma urealyticum* (previously called T-strain *Mycoplasma)* are the genera implicated as causes of reproductive failure. These organisms are characterized by their small size, their absence of a true cell wall, and their ability to grow in cell-free media.

Mycoplasma hominis and *U. ureolyticum* are commonly detected in the lower genitourinary tract of men and women. Investigators have noted a direct correlation between the prevalence of both organisms and sexual activity with different partners. Although the region of the genital tract most likely to be colonized by mycoplasmas is the vagina, there is sufficient evidence to suggest that lower genitourinary tract colonization can lead to upper tract infection involving the uterus and potentially the placenta and fetus.

Couples were treated with three regimens: doxycycline, 200 mg/day for one menstrual cycle; erythromycin, 250 mg every 6 hours for the duration of the pregnancy begun in the third month; and a combination of doxycycline and erythromycin. A 28-day course of doxycycline eradicated *U. urealyticum* from

87.6% of couples and *M. hominis* from 100% of couples. If couples were colonized with both organisms, only 61.3% of them were cleared with one course of doxycycline. A significant reduction in the rate of pregnancy loss was noted in all three treatment groups versus those who were not treated. It is important to consider that in this study, pregnancy loss was defined as spontaneous miscarriages, stillborn infants, premature infants who died, or term infants who died at birth. Possible association of improved outcome with other factors was not explored. Furthermore, the authors state that patients were not strictly randomized.

In summary, in a limited number of poorly controlled studies, women with recurrent pregnancy loss have been found to have a higher incidence of *M. hominis* or *U. urealyticum* colonization or infection than women with normal reproductive histories. A purposed pathophysiologic mechanism is that mycoplasmas ascend from the vagina, cross the placenta, and result in early fetal demise. There are a limited number of cases with microbiologic data to support the contention that infection with mycoplasmas is associated with sporadic cases of septic early spontaneous miscarriage. The existing data do not substantiate that Mycoplasma colonization cause's recurrent pregnancy loss or that eradication of colonization improves outcome.

Toxoplasmosis

Toxoplasma gondii is an obligate intracellular parasite. It may exist in three forms: the tachyzoite, the tissue cyst, and the oocyte. The reproductive cycle of this parasite is carried out in the cat, and oocytes are excreted in cat feces. The tachyzoites are invasive and persist intracellularly. The tissue cysts may also invade body tissues and are the chronic forms. Humans become infected by ingesting poorly cooked or raw meat of infected animals and by direct contact with cat feces, or feces-contaminated environment such as contaminated soil, vegetables, and barnyards. Once a person is infected, there is a parasitemia that is usually asymptomatic. The intact immune system then confers protection against parasites that invade body tissues.

Toxoplasmosis is a well-documented intrauterine pathogen. It can be associated with congenital infection when maternal infection occurs at any time during pregnancy. It is thought that maternal infection during the first trimester can result in intrauterine infection and fetal loss. A purported pathophysiologic mechanism for toxoplasmosis infection in pregnancy is that after maternal parasitemia occurs, the parasites reside in the placenta and may cross into the fetal space. Therefore, recurrent miscarriages caused by toxoplasmosis might occur if recurrent maternal parasitemias were demonstrated or if the parasites resided in the endometrium. However, the results of studies that attempt to establish toxoplasmosis as an etiology for habitual miscarriage are varied.

Investigators found that 9% of women with miscarriage were antibody-positive versus 7% of the control group. Furthermore, there was no difference in antibody status between sporadic and habitual aborters. In this study, the authors report considerable difficulty in isolating *T. gondii* from the endometrium, which is crucial to linking chronic Toxoplasma to recurrent miscarriage. Desmonts and Couvreur evaluated 378 pregnant women with high initial antibody titers or seroconversion during pregnancy. These investigators found that toxoplasmosis had no effect on pregnancy outcome of women who were previously antibody-positive. In summary, it appears that epidemiologic studies and some pathologic studies have associated Toxoplasma infection with sporadic pregnancy loss; however, data on recurrent pregnancy loss are anecdotal at best.

LISTERIA

Listeria monocytogenes is a gram-positive rod that may be found in various animal species, soil, and plants. It is a rare cause of sporadic human disease and has caused a few well-described, geographically isolated epidemics. Disease is most prevalent among the elderly, the immunocompromised, pregnant women, and newborn infants.

How Can I Suspect if I Had a Listeria Infection?

Maternal infection may be characterized by acute onset of fever or abdominal and back pain, or occasionally it may be asymptomatic. The newborn may be affected by early-onset disease presumed from maternal transmission during pregnancy. Both are associated with significant morbidity and mortality, with overall fatality rates in the 30% range.

Summary

Listeria may cause premature rupture of the fetal membranes and neonatal morbidity and mortality. The current belief, however is that *Listeria monocytogenes* is not an etiology for recurrent pregnancy loss.

CHLAMYDIA

Chlamydia trachomatis is an obligate intracellular bacterium that has specific phagocytic properties that allow this bacterium to infect its host. The predominant mode of transmission is sexual. There are 15 known serotypes of C. *trachomatis*, with strains D through K being the sexually transmitted types. The prevalence of C. *trachomatis* in the pregnant population is reported to be between 2% and 37%.

Several studies have attempted to determine if maternal Chlamydia infection is associated with adverse pregnancy outcome. A positive Chlamydia culture is correlated with more low-birth-weight infants and more premature rupture of the membranes.

Summary

Although stillbirth and neonatal death occurred in 33% of patients with positive Chlamydia cultures versus 3.4% in pregnancies of noninfected women, there has no association of positive Chlamydia infection and spontaneous miscarriages.

GROUP B STREPTOCOCCUS

Group B beta-hemolytic streptococci or *Streptococcus agalactiae* is a facultative gram-positive diplococcus. It has been suggested that group B streptococcus may infect the fetal membrane and result in spontaneous miscarriage in addition to adverse outcomes in later gestation. The number of mothers with positive group B streptococcus cultures is frequent. An ascending infection causes amnionitis and subsequent fetal infection. Stillbirth or deaths occur soon after birth between 18 and 27 weeks gestation.

Approximately 37% of pregnancies of mothers with positive group B streptococcus cervical cultures ended in spontaneous miscarriage, perinatal death, prematurity, and severe neonatal illness. Strong data from numerous pathology investigations suggest that group B streptococcus may cause sporadic spontaneous miscarriage via transplacental spread.

11

Hormones and Miscarriage

LUTEAL PHASE DEFECT

What is Luteal Phase Defect?

Luteal phase defect (LPD) refers to the development of immature secretory endometrium due to an inadequately functioning corpus luteum. Estimates of the incidence of LPD in women with reproductive failure ranges from 6.6% to 40%. The diagnosis is made following two consecutive endometrial biopsies "out of phase" by 3 or more days. Diagnosis of luteal insufficiency has also been attempted via measurement of serum or urinary levels of progesterone and its metabolites. Wide fluctuations of progesterone levels during the luteal phase, however, limit the reliability of this approach.

The term *luteal phase defect* is often used to describe the clinical condition of corpus luteum insufficiency. A LPD refers to a relative deficiency in the secretion of progesterone by the corpus luteum. The life span of the normal corpus luteum is between 11 and 16 days. Luteal phase defects are often subclassified according to the relative amount or duration of progesterone production. The *inadequate luteal phase* refers to a luteal phase of normal length with lower than normal progesterone secretion. The *short luteal phase* refers to a shortening of the interval between ovulation and the onset of menses to 10 days or less.

The incidence of LPD as a pathologic condition is difficult to determine. This is largely due to the lack of uniform diagnostic criteria in the various epidemiologic reports. In addition, there is a limited amount of data to address the incidence of LPD in the "normal" population. Davis recently reported that the incidence of LPD in normal fertile women was 6.6%. The incidence of LPD as a cause for infertility has been reported to be between 3% and 20%. Because the majority of series estimate the incidence to be between 3% and 10%, LPD may not represent a clinically significant cause of infertility.

In contrast to patients with infertility, patients with recurrent pregnancy loss have a significantly higher incidence of LPDs. The reported incidence of LPD among patients with recurrent pregnancy loss appears to vary between 23% and 60%. Luteal Phase Defect is felt to occur in many women who are menstruating regularly or irregularly, but not ovulating optimally. Thus, an evaluation for LPD should be considered in all patients with recurrent pregnancy loss.

What Causes Luteal Phase Defect?

One possible cause of LPD is hyperprolactinemia; the probable mechanism is an inhibition of pulsatile gonadotropin releasing hormone secretion by the hypothalamus, although direct ovarian effects of hyperprolactinemia cannot be excluded. Correction of luteal phase deficiency with bromocriptine should be attempted in these cases.

There is no general consensus regarding the pathophysiology of LPD. The causes of LPD seem to involve a wide range of hypothalamic, pituitary, ovarian, or endometrial factors. The most common underlying mechanism appears to be an impairment of folliculogenesis. Women with LPDs have significantly lower serum follicle-stimulating hormone (FSH) levels compared to normal women. A relative decrease in serum FSH levels may result in a decreased number of LH receptors and an inadequate production of progesterone by the corpus luteum. The clinical association of weight loss, strenuous exercise, and the menarche with LPD further supports an etiologic role for hypothalamic dysfunction.

A minority of cases of LPD may be due to abnormal ovarian or uterine responsiveness. In the perimenopausal woman, the development of irregular menstrual cycles may be due to a LPD. The decreased production of progesterone by the perimenopausal ovary may be the result of inadequate folliculogenesis due to a waning number of primordial follicles. Pathologic conditions involving the ovary, such as endometriosis, may also interfere with normal follicular development and result in decreased progesterone production.

How Do You Diagnose LPD?

There are no uniform diagnostic criteria for LPD. Thus, a major goal in the field of reproductive endocrinology is to standardize the diagnostic criteria. There is still considerable debate over the optimal method for timing and interpreting the endometrial biopsy. Despite these controversies, all patients with recurrent pregnancy loss should be evaluated for LPD. A summary of the advantages and disadvantages of the various diagnostic tests is presented in Table 1.

Table 1. Diagnostic Methods for Luteal Phase Defect

DIAGNOSTIC METHODS	CRITERIA	ADVANTAGES	DISADVANTAGES
Basal body temperature recording	Luteal phase <11 days	Simplicity	Lacks both sensitivity and specificity
Progesterone Determinations	Midluteal concentration <14 ng/ml	Objective	Misinterpretation due to short-term fluctuations in serum levels
Endometrial biopsy	Histology >2 days out of phase with known day of ovulation	Identifies abnormalities resulting from deficient corpus luteum	Discomfort; requires expertise in histopathology; expense

How Does Progesterone Assist With the Maintenance of Pregnancy?

Researchers studied the effects of luteectomy and progesterone replacement in pregnant patients. They concluded that the production of progesterone by the corpus luteum is essential for the maintenance of pregnancy up until the seventh week of gestation. The importance of progesterone is further supported by the discovery that the antiprogestin RU-486 can effectively terminate early pregnancy.

Although progesterone is known to be important for implantation and the maintenance of early pregnancy, its physiology and biochemistry at the cellular level remain poorly understood. Women with LPD may have decreased glycogen content in their endometrium leading to lower implantation success.

The field of endometrial protein biology is rapidly emerging as an important component of the implantation process. There are a large number of progestin associated and progestin dependent endometrial proteins, several of which appear to be clinically significant. The endometrial protein, progestagen-associated endometrial protein (PEP), is secreted in increasing quantities from the proliferative phase through the early stages of pregnancy. Significantly lower levels of PEP in women with LPD. Similar to PEP, endometrial Prolactin production is progesterone-dependent and appears to be decreased in patients with LPD.

The role of progesterone in the maintenance of early pregnancy may be partially due to its immunosuppressive activity. During normal pregnancy, the developing embryo is immunologically protected from rejection by the maternal immune systems. An additional mechanism of action for progesterone is its ability to cause smooth muscle relaxation. During early pregnancy, progesterone appears to contribute to the maintenance of a quiescent myometrium. The muscle relaxant properties of progesterone may be mediated by the inhibition of uterine prostaglandin. In addition, because uterine Prolactin stimulates myometrial contractility, the muscle relaxant properties of progesterone may also be partially mediated by the inhibition of myometrial prolactin production.

Basal Body Temperature

The basal body temperature (BBT) chart is notoriously inaccurate for the diagnosis of LPD. Although a biphasic temperature chart strongly suggests an ovulatory cycle, a monophasic pattern does not necessarily indicate an ovulatory disorder. Documented hormonal evidence of ovulation in approximately 75% of monophasic cycles. In addition, there is no correlation between the absolute magnitude of the temperature rise and the presence or absence of a LPD.

The BBT chart may be helpful in determining the length of the luteal phase. A luteal phase of less than 11 days (short luteal phase) appears to be associated with an increased incidence of LPD. Andrews initially suggested that the length of the luteal phase be considered in the diagnosis of LPD. The subsequent studies of Downs and Gibson and Lenton confirmed the significant correlation between mean luteal phase length and the presence or absence of a LPD. Andrews also suggested that the rate of the temperature rise be considered in the diagnosis of LPD; however, Downs and Gibson found no correlation between the rate of the temperature rise and the incidence of LPD. These authors concluded that a slow temperature rise (the staircase effect") may reflect variable central nervous system responsiveness but does not indicate a LPD.

The major disadvantage of the BBT chart in the diagnosis of LPD is its lack of sensitivity. Although a short luteal phase is highly suggestive of LPD, a normal luteal phase length does not rule out significant corpus luteum dysfunction. In fact, the majority of patients with LPD do not have a short luteal phase.

Serum Progesterone

A single midluteal serum progesterone level greater than 5 ng/ml is indirect evidence of ovulation. It is generally accepted that a midluteal progesterone level of greater than 14 ng/ml is associated with adequate corpus luteum function. Although a single midluteal progesterone determination offers a practical and cost-effective approach to the evaluation of LPD, there are limited conclusive data to support these recommendations. In fact, other investigators have demonstrated significant overlap among single serum progesterone levels obtained from LPD patients and normal controls. In addition, there is a poor correlation between a single serum progesterone level and the endometrial biopsy in the evaluation of LPD. The difficulty encountered in the interpretation of a single midluteal serum progesterone level may be due to the pulsatile nature of progesterone secretion.

Over the years, considerable efforts to improve the diagnostic accuracy of serum progesterone levels in the evaluation of LPD have focused on increasing the frequency of blood sampling. Because there is general agreement that the majority of cases of LPD are associated with decreased progesterone secretion, it is not surprising that increasing the frequency of blood sampling increases the diagnostic accuracy of serum progesterone determinations. Unfortunately, there is no consensus regarding the optimal number and timing of multiple progesterone determinations. Moreover, the absolute level of progesterone production that accurately reflects normal luteal function has not been determined. The major disadvantages of multiple blood sampling include the inconvenience and expense.

Endometrial Biopsy

Endometrial biopsy is considered the standard diagnostic test for the evaluation of LPD. The endometrial biopsy not only identifies inadequate progesterone production by the corpus luteum but also identifies abnormal endometrial responsiveness. As previously mentioned, the optimal criteria for diagnosing LPD remain controversial. Both midluteal serum progesterone levels and late luteal endometrial histology should be assessed in the evaluation of LPD. The most widely accepted criteria include endometrial dating, which lags behind the time in the cycle by more than 2 days when derived retrospectively in two separate cycles. A single normal endometrial biopsy is often termed *in phase* and is usually considered sufficient to exclude the diagnosis of LPD. An abnormal biopsy is generally required in two separate cycles to make the diagnosis of LPD because an isolated "out-of-phase" biopsy is not uncommon in normally fertile women. The accuracy of the endometrial biopsy as a diagnostic test is highly dependent on the experience of the pathologist interpreting the histologic specimen.

Traditionally, the endometrial biopsy is performed 2 to 3 days prior to the time of the expected menses. If the biopsy is performed prior to the 25th day, there is an increased rate of false-negative results. In patients with slightly irregular menstrual cycles, accurately timing the endometrial biopsy is often difficult. An accurate interpretation of the endometrial biopsy should be based on days since ovulation rather than onset of menses. It has similarly demonstrated an improved accuracy for dating the endometrial biopsy based on serum luteinizing hormone determinations when compared with subsequent menses.

A rapid and sensitive serum pregnancy test should be offered to the patient immediately prior to the biopsy in an attempt to prevent the interruption of an early pregnancy. However, despite a negative pregnancy test, inadvertent disruption of an early pregnancy remains a possibility. Several studies have analyzed the effects of performing an endometrial biopsy in the cycle of conception. The incidence of performing a biopsy following conception has been estimated to be between 0.2% and 6.7%. Fortunately, the likelihood of removing or interrupting the implantation site appears to be quite low (<2% for pregnant patients and <0.067% for the entire biopsy population). The majority of these studies indicate there is no increase in the incidence of miscarriage, prematurity, or congenital anomalies.

There is increasing use of ultrasound for the diagnosis of abnormal endometrial responsiveness. Preovulatory qualitative patterns of endometrial associated with quantitative thickness have been associated with serum mid-luteal progesterone levels for increased appreciation of this diagnosis. The benefit of this assessment is the reduction of pain associated with a non-invasive procedure.

What is the Treatment of LPD?

Therapy for LPD is hormonal. Some investigators have demonstrated success with natural progesterone supplementation in the treatment of this disorder.

Alternatively, ovulation induction may be administered in the follicular phase. Progesterone and clomiphene have equivalent success rates in the treatment of LPD. Once hormonal therapy is initiated, a follow-up endometrial biopsy, pelvic ultrasound or assessment of a serum progesterone level may be performed to document correction of Luteal Phase Defect.

A variety of medical therapies have been reported for the treatment of LPD (Table 2). This is not surprising, because the pathophysiology of LPD appears to be multifactorial. Whenever possible, identifiable causes of LPD should be specifically treated. In the absence of a specific cause, a variety of therapeutic approaches should be considered. The treatment options include stimulation of folliculogenesis, stimulation of luteal function, and luteal phase progesterone supplementation. The two most commonly employed therapies are clomiphene citrate and progesterone. The various therapeutic agents are largely recommended based on data from clinical series. A significant improvement in pregnancy outcome follows treatment of LPD among patients with a history of recurrent pregnancy loss.

Table 2. Treatment Options for Luteal Phase Defect

MEDICATION	DOSE
Clomiphene citrate	50 mg PO days 5-9
Progesterone	12.5-25 mg vaginally twice-daily
	12.5-25 mg IM every day beginning the day after ovulation
Bromocriptine	2.5 mg PO hid
Human Chorionic Gonadotropin	2500 IU IM every 3 days for 3 doses to begin 3 days after ovulation
Gonadotropins	75—225 IU every day

Clomiphene Citrate

The rationale for clomiphene therapy is that normal luteal function requires optimal follicular development and clomiphene stimulates folliculogenesis. Several studies in support of this hypothesis have demonstrated that clomiphene augments gonadotropin secretion and increases luteal progesterone production in women with LPD.

The recommended starting dose for clomiphene is 50 mg for 5 days. Clomiphene is administered on cycle days 3 to 7 or 5 to 9. The majority of patients (84%) conceive during the first three treatment cycles. Once normal endometrial maturation was obtained, pregnancies occurred at rates comparable to those in the normal population.

Although the dose of clomiphene is often increased if the endometrial biopsy remains "out of phase," the inability of clomiphene to correct a LPD may be due to its anti-estrogenic activity at the level of the uterus. Some authors regard the use of clomiphene for LPD as inappropriate owing to its peripheral anti-estrogenic activity. Clomiphene has been shown to decrease endometrial estrogen and progesterone receptor content. Several studies have demonstrated that the anti-estrogenic activity of clomiphene may adversely affect the quantity and quality of the cervical mucus as well as paradoxically cause LPD. Therefore, in addition to repeating the endometrial biopsy, a postcoital test is often recommended during clomiphene therapy.

Progesterone

The rationale behind progesterone therapy is simply supplementing inadequate progesterone levels with the natural hormone. The results from a large number of clinical series suggest that progesterone supplementation for LPD may be beneficial in patients with recurrent pregnancy loss. Progesterone therapy has also been shown to correct abnormal endometrial maturation in 80% of infertility patients with LPDs, and crude pregnancy rates in infertility patients have ranged from 50% to 80%.

Progesterone therapy should begin 2 to 3 days after the LH surge, because earlier administration may inhibit ovulation. Progesterone supplementation may be administered as a vaginal suppository twice a day, or as an intramuscular injection daily. Progesterone therapy is continued until the onset of menses or if pregnancy ensues through 8-9 weeks gestation. Although controversial, synthetic progestagens should be avoided owing to their potential teratogenic and luteolytic effects. The safety of progesterone appears to be well documented, and there is no evidence for an increased risk of congenital malformations.

Human Chorionic Gonadotropin

The rationale behind therapy with human chorionic gonadotropin (HCG) is to stimulate the corpus luteum to produce progesterone, because HCG is biologically similar to luteinizing hormone and will stimulate the production of progesterone via luteinizing hormone receptors in the corpus luteum. Most investigators do not advocate HCG as a primary therapy for LPD. Animal studies suggest that the timing of HCG administration is critical. Early luteal administration may promote atresia, and late luteal administration results in a brief and attenuated progesterone response. There are virtually no human studies to address the efficacy of HCG therapy. It has been reported that HCG supplementation is less effective than progesterone replacement in reversing a LPD. The recommended doses are arbitrary and range from 1500 to 5000 IU every 2 to 5 days after the LH surge for approximately 12 days. Because of its long half-life, administration of HCG interferes with a urine or serum pregnancy test for approximately 7 days after the last injection.

Elevated Prolactin

Bromocriptine should be considered the drug of choice for patients with LPD secondary to hyperprolactinemia. Finally, several investigators have reported on the potential usefulness of gonadotropin therapy and pulsatile gonadotropin releasing hormone in the treatment of LPD.

Summary of Luteal Phase Deficiency

The epidemiologic studies of recurrent pregnancy loss seem to suggest an etiologic role for LPD. The majority of LPDs seem to result from an impairment of follicular development. The mechanism of recurrent pregnancy loss in patients with LPDs is not known; however, future studies are likely to confirm the importance of progesterone-dependent proteins during implantation and early pregnancy. An evaluation for LPD should be considered in all patients with recurrent pregnancy loss. The BBT chart may identify a short luteal phase. The endometrial biopsy is considered the standard diagnostic test for LPD. The optimal methods for timing and interpreting the endometrial biopsy remain controversial. At the present time, the most widely accepted diagnostic criteria include endometrial dating, which lags behind the time in the cycle by more than 2 days when derived retrospectively in two separate cycles. A variety of medical therapies have been reported for the treatment of LPD. The two most commonly employed therapies, clomiphene citrate and progesterone, seem to be equally efficacious.

THYROID DISEASE

Hypothyroidism has been reported as a cause of pregnancy loss. These conclusions are derived from retrospective review of pregnancies in patients with and without thyroid disease. It remains unclear, however, whether thyroid disease is actually an etiologic factor or simply an associated coincidental finding. The diagnosis of hypothyroidism is made via the thyroid-stimulating hormone (TSH) assay. Although the yield is low, thyroid function testing is generally recommended in the evaluation of a patient with habitual miscarriage.

DIABETES MELLITUS

There are no studies implicating subclinical or adequately controlled diabetes mellitus as a cause of recurrent miscarriage. However, women with poorly controlled insulin-dependent diabetes have a 2-to 3-fold higher rate of spontaneous miscarriage than do nondiabetic women. For a patient with second-or third-trimester pregnancy loss or clinical signs of diabetes, an investigation of carbohydrate tolerance is warranted. However, for most women with first-trimester spontaneous miscarriages, a routine glucose-tolerance test is not indicated.

Review of Miscarriage and Diabetes

Spontaneous miscarriages among diabetic pregnancies, which is not significantly different from the spontaneous miscarriage rates recently published in nondiabetic patients. The review did not find convincing evidence of a difference in the risk of spontaneous miscarriage among diabetics when mean maternal age, disease duration, White classification, frequency of miscarriage in previous pregnancies, smoking history, and use of medications were considered as separate risk factors. There was no difference in the risk of spontaneous miscarriage (10%) among gestational diabetics. However, there was a suggestion of a relation between spontaneous miscarriage and elevated glycosylated hemoglobin level

(Hb A_1), which is a measure of average glycemic concentration during the proceeding 4 to 8 weeks.

Recurrent Miscarriage

The frequency of repetitive spontaneous miscarriages among diabetic women is not increased. There is no significant difference in the incidence of recurrent miscarriage among insulin-requiring diabetics (6.9%) and nondiabetic controls (5.7%). Researchers have found that the risk of spontaneous miscarriage was 16% in both diabetic women and nondiabetic controls.

A study describing the relationship between the level of Hb A_1 in the first trimester and spontaneous miscarriage in insulin-requiring diabetics has been conducted. Thirty-five percent of patients were in poor glycemic control with Hb A_1 levels greater than nine standard deviations above the mean for a nondiabetic population. They found that the risk of spontaneous miscarriage was significantly increased at greater than nine standard deviations above the mean and the risk of major congenital malformation was significantly increased at greater than 12 standard deviations above the mean. White classification did not correlate with the risk for spontaneous miscarriage. The risk for spontaneous miscarriage in the entire series of diabetics was 17.2%. Women with a Hb A_1 less than or equal to nine standard deviations above the mean had a risk of spontaneous miscarriage of approximately 10%, similar to that reported for the general population. At higher levels of Hb A_1, the risk of spontaneous miscarriage ranged from 25% to 38%.

The cause of increased spontaneous miscarriages in diabetics with poor glucose control is not clear. It may be due to mild metabolic abnormalities associated with maternal diabetes. Because there is a high incidence of major malformations among spontaneous abortuses and poor glycemic control is associated with an increased risk of malformation, the excess risk of loss may be due to a high number of hyperglycemia-induced major malformations in this population. In vitro experiments by several authors have demonstrated the adverse effects of hyperglycemia and other metabolic abnormalities of diabetes on cell growth and development.

Summary of Diabetes and Pregnancy Loss

Diabetic women with good or moderately good glycemic control are at no increased risk for spontaneous miscarriage above the risk for the general population (10% to 20%). Women with poor glycemic control, defined as glycosylated hemoglobin at least six to nine standard deviations above the mean, are at increased risk for spontaneous miscarriage. This risk is probably due to increased numbers of malformed embryos, severe hyperglycemia, and as yet not well-defined metabolic abnormalities in diabetic gravidas. In the absence of persistent or recurrent poor glycemic control, diabetes is not a cause of recurrent early pregnancy loss.

I do not believe that glucose tolerance testing should be performed as part of the evaluation of pregnancy loss unless there is other evidence that the patient may be diabetic. The clinician should be suspicious if glucosuria is present and fasting blood glucose is greater than 115 mg/dl or random blood glucose is 160 mg/dl or greater.

POLYCYSTIC OVARY (PCO) SYNDROME

It is well known that PCO can cause menstrual disorders ranging from no menstrual periods (amenorrhea) to dysfunctional uterine bleeding, plus hirsutism and infertility. In addition, the unopposed estrogen secretion can increase endometrial cancer risk by 3-fold and perhaps breast cancer risk by 3-to 4-fold. Anovulatory women who are overweight, hyperandrogenic, and hyperinsulinemic should also have a heightened risk of diabetes.

Patients with PCO appear to have an increased risk of spontaneous miscarriage. This has been attributed to elevated levels of luteinizing hormone (LH) that may produce an adverse environment for the oocyte, perhaps even inducing premature maturation and completion of the first meiotic division. Tonic hypersecretion of LH occurs only in women with PCO. While an elevated LH value in the presence of a low or low-normal follicle stimulating hormone (FSH) level is diagnostic, the condition is often evident through clinical presentation alone. However, 20% to 40% of patients with PCO do not have elevated LH levels.

Consideration should be given to LH suppression before attempting treatment. Ovulation induction can be achieved using clomiphene citrate, human menopausal gonadotropins (hMG), or pure FSH. Pituitary desensitization or down-regulation with gonadotropin-releasing hormone (GNRH) prior to the use of FSH or hMG may improve pregnancy outcome, and is now employed by most assisted-reproduction centers.

Treatment of insulin resistance often seen with PCO has been performed. Agents such as glucophage have been used preconceptually with diet and weight loss to improve pregnancy outcomes in these patients. Ongoing studies are being performed to clarify their role in decreased reproductive loss!

12

Reproductive Immunology

AUTOIMMUNITY AND RECURRENT PREGNANCY LOSS

Several autoimmune diseases have been associated with recurrent pregnancy loss. Among these autoimmune diseases, systemic lupus erythematosus (SLE) and the antiphospholipid (APL) syndrome have been closely associated with pregnancy loss.

Systemic Lupus Erythematosus

There are now three prospective studies of pregnancy in women with well-documented SLE. The overall pregnancy loss rate (spontaneous miscarriages and fetal deaths) ranged from 22% to 30%, slightly higher than the 10% clinical pregnancy loss rate expected among normal pregnant women aged 25 to 34 years. One study included a control group of normal pregnant women and found that there was a significantly greater rate of pregnancy loss before 20 weeks' gestation in SLE patients (5.7% versus 16%). None of these studies controlled for the effect of previous miscarriage or fetal death in their patients with SLE. The majority of fetal losses in women with SLE are predicted by the presence of antiphospholipid antibodies.

Subclinical Autoimmunity

Autoimmunity is not confined to the clinically obvious. Small proportions of "normal" asymptomatic individuals have circulating autoantibodies and are generally considered to have a subclinical autoimmune "diathesis." The long-term implications of this are not known, although it has recently become apparent that some of these women have recurrent pregnancy loss or fetal death as the only manifestation of their autoimmune condition. Several different autoantibodies may be relevant, but again APL has been the most strongly implicated.

THROMBOPHILIAS

The Antiphospholipid Syndrome (APS)

Antiphospholipid (APL) are autoantibodies with specificity for negatively charged phospholipids. Two APL are recognized: lupus anticoagulant (LA) and anticardiolipin antibody (ACL). LA and ACL are the most important clinically, having been associated with thrombosis (blood clotting) and recurrent pregnancy loss.

Antiphospholipid antibodies are formed after the mother's immune system is exposed to the products of conception. The antiphospholipid antibody syndrome can be primary or secondary. Women who have antiphospholipid antibodies demonstrate a hypercoagulable state within the placenta, and tend to abort in the first or second trimesters. This occurs via platelet membrane damage, endothelial wall damage, inhibition of prostacyclin, and inability to activate protein C. Furthermore, antiphospholipid antibodies inhibit the formation of cells that compose the placenta. Fortunately, therapy is available with blood thinners (anticoagulation). Antiphospholipid levels can change over time, so this test needs to be repeated from time to time.

Antiphospholipid Syndrome and Recurrent Pregnancy Loss

The risk of pregnancy loss in women with APS appears to be fairly high. For women with this syndrome, the chance of a successful untreated pregnancy is only about 10%. The poorest outcomes were among women with previous fetal death and/or high levels of ACL. Women with previous fetal death and high levels of ACL suffered a fetal loss rate of 70%. For any level of ACL, a history of previous pregnancy loss more than doubled the risk of fetal loss in the next pregnancy. Recent studies of pregnant women show that some women with significant levels of APL, but without prior manifestations of the syndrome, have live infants. In this sense, APL is like ANAs: the presence of the antibodies alone does not predict clinical disease. Not surprisingly, the highest prevalence of APL is found among patients with autoimmune disease. Between 6% and 24% of patients with Systemic Lupus Erythematosis (SLE) have LA; up to 40% have measurable levels of ACL. This probably explains some of the increased fetal loss noted in lupus pregnancies. However, it is important to realize that not all of fetal losses in lupus pregnancies are associated with APL.

How often is the APS an explanation for recurrent pregnancy loss?

10% of patients with unexplained recurrent pregnancy loss had LA. Studies of ACL and pregnancy loss found that 11% to 42% of women with unexplained recurrent pregnancy loss had ACL. This prevalence is sufficient to recommend testing all patients with recurrent pregnancy loss or fetal death for APL, especially because the assays are relatively inexpensive and the condition appears to be treatable.

Among women with APS, at least 30% of the pregnancy losses occur as fetal deaths in the second trimester. Over 90% of patients with APS have had at least one fetal death, indicating the importance placed on determining the absence or presence of a fetus in women with a pregnancy loss.

How common are Antiphospholipids (APL)?

The overall frequency of APL in the general population is unknown, but several studies provide prevalence data for selected populations. The prevalence of ACL among normal nonpregnant controls is about 2%. ACL is detected more frequently than LA, probably because of the greater sensitivity of the ACL assays.

What is the Pathophysiology of Autoimmune Pregnancy Loss?

The relatively few studies that address the pathophysiology of autoimmune-associated pregnancy loss have focused on patients with SLE, APL, or both. The pathology immediately responsible for pregnancy loss appears to be a necrotizing vasculopathy at the maternal-placental interface. This same vasculopathy has been described in the placentas of women with APL and pregnancy loss.

Plasma or immunoglobulin (IgG) fractions from patients with LA have been shown to inhibit vascular endothelial prostacyclin production. It has been proposed that this leads to vascular damage due to vasoconstriction and then thrombosis. It has also been suggested that APL inhibits prostacyclin generation from vascular tissues by binding to endothelial cell membranes.

What Treatment is Available?

Aggressive treatment of patients with APL and previous pregnancy loss may improve the chance of delivering a viable infant. Women with LA have had successful pregnancy outcomes when treated with prednisone and low-dose aspirin.

Experience suggests that treatment with corticosteroids and low-dose aspirin is beneficial but certainly does not guarantee success. Prednisone, especially in the high doses used, is a potentially dangerous drug with serious adverse effects.

The problems associated with high-dose steroid therapy, coupled with the finding that thrombosis is a key feature of women with APL, have led to the use of heparin (a blood thinner) and low dose aspirin therapy during pregnancy. Studies have shown greater than 70% delivery of viable infants when heparin and low dose aspirin have been instituted.

When is IVIG a useful treatment?

Another potentially useful treatment for APL-associated pregnancy loss is intravenous immunoglobulin (IVIG). The lack of serious adverse effects makes this therapy attractive, although it is very expensive.

Recently, another mechanism for immunologically mediated pregnancy loss has been elucidated. Patients with high levels of CD56+CD19+ natural killer (NK) cells or high levels of CD5+CD19+ cytotoxic B-cells are at risk for pregnancy loss due to cellular immune mediated mechanisms. Recent studies have demonstrated the efficacy of intravenous immunoglobulin G (IVIG) in such cases.

Systemic Lupus Erythematosus and Lupus Anticoagulant

Autoimmune conditions such as systemic lupus erythematosus (SLE) are associated with an increased risk of pregnancy loss usually in association with antiphospholipid antibodies (APL), from 7% to 30% of women with SLE have APL. Otherwise healthy women with APL are also at greater risk of recurrent pregnancy loss. Three types of APL are of clinical relevance: lupus anticoagulant (LA), anticardiolipin antibodies (ACL), and biologically false-positive serologic results for syphilis (FP-STS). The presence of APL has been linked to several medical conditions, including pregnancy loss, arterial and venous thromboses, autoimmune thrombocytopenia, and autoimmune hemolytic anemia. Some 80% of patients with APL and fetal death show evidence of placental blood clot formation and death of the placenta where the blood flow was blocked (infarction).

Systemic lupus erythematosus is associated with second-trimester pregnancy loss. Laboratory markers for this alloimmune disorder include ANA, lupus anticoagulant, and ACL. Antinuclear antibodies directed at various nuclear components are found in greater than 95% of patients with SLE. These antibodies probably have little direct role in recurrent pregnancy loss. The ACL, measured by enzyme-linked immunosorbent assay, is directed at phospholipids and is found in 40% to 60% of patients with SLE. Several authors have suggested that a high ACL titer is the most sensitive and specific predictor of poor pregnancy outcome.

The lupus anticoagulant, a heterogeneous group of immunoglobulins directed at membrane phospholipids, has also been strongly associated with recurrent fetal loss and thrombosis. In fact, recurrent pregnancy loss is often the initial presenting symptom in women subsequently found to have the lupus anticoagulant. This antibody complex is commonly present in patients with connective tissue disorders as well as in association with numerous other systemic diseases. Although only 5% to 15% of patients with SLE have the lupus anticoagulant, 40% of patients with the lupus anticoagulant have systemic lupus.

Although the lupus anticoagulant causes prolongation of various clotting parameters, it is commonly associated with a hypercoagulable state. With regard to the paradoxical effect, lupus anticoagulant has procoagulant properties that are thought to inhibit fibrinolysis by impairing phospholipid-induced activation of protein C, a cofactor in the fibrinolytic cascade. In addition, it probably causes increased platelet aggregation and adhesiveness by nonspecifically injuring platelet and endothelial phospholipid membranes. This is thought to result in recurrent systemic thrombosis, which during pregnancy may lead to infarction of the placental circulation.

Therapeutic intervention has been advocated for women with anticardiolipin or lupus anticoagulant who experience repeated pregnancy loss. Corticosteroids (with or without low-dose aspirin), aspirin, heparin, and gamma-globulin therapy have all been tried, but more prospective controlled, randomized studies demonstrating a clear advantage to these agents needs to be performed. Recent studies using therapeutic levels of heparin and low dose aspirin have shown promising results.

Major Histocompatibility Antigens

All fetuses possess antigens foreign to the mother, and yet survive pregnancy without rejection. The lack of classic human leukocyte antigen (HLA) on trophoblastic tissue suggests that trophoblast is immunologically inert, with an important protective role. Active modulation of the maternal immune system may also protect the developing embryo.

Earlier studies suggested that parental HLA heterogeneity was important for successful reproduction, but recent research fails to confirm that such heterogeneity serves to maintain human pregnancy. Therefore, testing couples for HLA sharing is no longer recommended for routine evaluation of recurrent miscarriage. Recent studies have shown no relationship between the degree of HLA incompatibility and the incidence of successful pregnancy outcome.

SUMMARY

Women with recurrent pregnancy loss often pose a particularly vexing problem for the clinician. Often, these women have delayed childbearing and are extremely motivated to achieve a normal term pregnancy. A conventional evaluation, including hysterosalpingography, luteal phase endometrial biopsy, and parental karyotyping, will identify an etiology for pregnancy loss in up to one half of patients. New data indicate that these women should be tested for the presence of APL, particularly if they have experienced a fetal death. Current treatment regimens appear to improve pregnancy outcome.

The use of low-dose aspirin (82 mg/day) and prednisolone in patients with APL during pregnancy is associated with a fetal survival rate of more than 50%. Alternatively, the use of heparin can improve outcome in 70% of these pregnancies. It should be noted that APL may be present in normal pregnancies, and patients with recurrent miscarriage may succeed without any treatment in subsequent pregnancies. However, both heparin and low dose aspirin therapy may be associated with increased risks for and severity of bleeding. Because the potential for bleeding exists with heparin and aspirin, the risks and benefits of anticoagulation therapy to improve success rates must be carefully assessed.

PART IV
ART—New Horizons

13

Assisted Reproductive Technology

At least one in ten couples of reproductive age are affected by infertility. Tubal disease, ovulatory defects, endometriosis, and abnormal sperm physiology are the most common causes of failure to conceive.

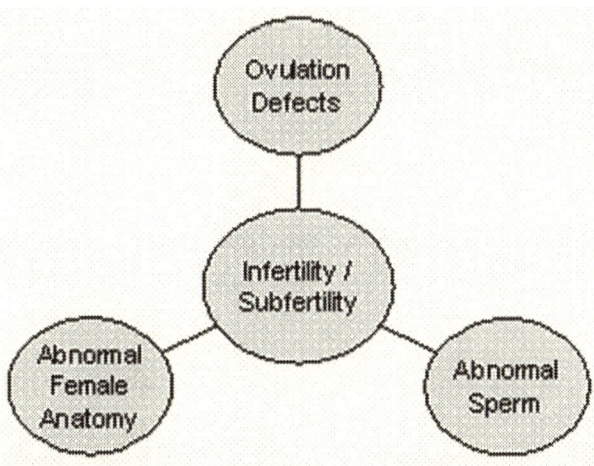

Many of these disorders can be treated successfully with surgery, ovulation induction or intrauterine insemination, but in selected cases or with long standing intractable infertility, assisted reproductive technology becomes the treatment of choice. In Table 1 are listed the commonly used acronyms in the assisted reproductive technology literature.

Table 1
Commonly used acronyms for assisted reproductive technology

IVF	In-vitro fertilization
GIFT	Gamete intrafallopian transfer
ZIFT	Zygote intrafallopian transfer
TET	Tubal embryo transfer
ICSI	Intracytoplasmic sperm injection
COS	Controlled ovarian stimulation
IUI	Intrauterine insemination

Brief History

A number of investigators throughout the twentieth century have contributed to the detailed knowledge of the mammalian reproductive cycle. As reviewed by Edwards, studies of human ovulation, fertilization and embryonic growth, coupled with technical advances in laparoscopy and pelvic ultrasound, have made the advances in assisted human conception possible. Edwards excised human oocytes from ovarian biopsies, matured them *in-vitro*, and studied human meiosis and fertilization.

Oocyte culture and fertilization, using washed ejaculated spermatozoa and oocytes matured *in-vitro*, was achieved in 1969 using a simple culture medium that was highly efficient in sustaining hamster fertilization *in-vitro*. Success in humans was achieved ten years later when Steptoe and Edwards reported the first live born conceived by *in-vitro* fertilization (IVF) in 1978. This pregnancy involved aspiration of a single oocyte during a natural cycle and replacement of a cleaving embryo during the natural luteal phase.

Pregnancy success increased to more than 25% when three embryos were replaced. Advancements in ovulation induction included the use of gonadotropin-releasing hormone (GnRH) analogs to achieve pituitary down-regulation before stimulation with human menopausal gonadotropins. The first successful pregnancy following gamete intrafallopian transfer was reported in 1984, and successful variations of that technique, including zygote intrafallopian transfer (ZIFT) and tubal embryo transfer (TET), were reported in 1988. Embryo cryopreservation and transfer of thawed human embryos resulted in the birth of twins and singletons.

Another important technical advance of the 1980's was the widespread use of ultrasound for follicular monitoring and its application in 1984 to transvaginal ultrasound-guided oocyte aspiration. From these advances, insemination of oocyte results in fertilization with a high degree of success in all but extreme forms of male infertility, and even in the most severe male-factor cases, microinjection of spermatozoa into the cytoplasm of the egg (ICSI) offers new hope.

IN-VITRO FERTILIZATION AND EMBRYO TRANSFER (IVF-ET)

Indications

Although originally developed as a treatment for tubal factor infertility, indications for IVF have expanded and now include endometriosis, male-factor and unexplained infertility. Tubal disease accounts for about 25% of infertility. In moderate or severe cases of tubal disease, surgical repair is associated with extremely low pregnancy rates. Failure of prior tuboplasty, absence of both fallopian tubes, and the more severe cases of tubal pathology are the most frequent indications for IVF.

Male-factor infertility accounts for up to 40% of infertility; therefore a semen analysis is crucial to any initial infertility evaluation. According to the World Health Organization, male subfertility is defined as sperm density of $< 20 \times 10^6$ per mL, motility of less than 40%, and less than 60% morphologically normal spermatozoa.

Pelvic endometriosis refractory to medical or surgical therapy accounts for 25-35% of women undergoing IVF procedures. IVF is usually recommended one to two years after previous unsuccessful medical or surgical therapy, and the prognosis depends on the severity and extent of the endometriotic lesions as well as patient age and duration of infertility.

Unexplained infertility is found in about 10% of couples despite a thorough evaluation, including normal semen analysis, ovulation documentation, luteal phase assessment, laparoscopy and negative antisperm antibody assay. Treatment for these women often is empirical and includes ovulation prediction, timed intrauterine insemination, superovulation with human menopausal gonadotropins followed by intrauterine insemination, and ultimately by IVF, GIFT or related procedures.

Ovarian Stimulation Protocol

With *in-vitro* fertilization, pregnancy rates improve when multiple embryos are replaced; hence, controlled ovarian hyperstimulation currently is used to yield multiple eggs and embryos.

In 1982, Drs. Howard and Georgeanna Jones established IVF pregnancies using hMG. This led to almost a doubling of the success rates of IVF due to a higher quantity of oocytes retrieved. However, because of premature LH surges, the incidence of treatment cycle cancellation remained as high as 30-35%. Because GnRH agonists (GnRHa) suppress bioactive LH, it was hypothesized that pre-treatment with GnRHa followed by concomitant GnRHa and hMG therapy would prevent a premature LH surge and might also enhance multiple follicle development in poor responders. This was indeed the case, and an improved response was demonstrated in previously poor responders treated with a GnRHa (leuprolide acetate) plus hMG. This combination resulted in enhanced oocyte yield, decreased cycle cancellation, and increased pregnancy rates.

Most centers still favor a "long" GnRHa protocol that involves luteal phase down-regulation before hMG administration. A GnRHa, such as leuprolide 1 mg per day subcutaneously, is given before ovulation induction with gonadotropins to maintain a relatively hypogonadotropic state with respect to endogenous gonadotropin secretion. The GnRHa is given beginning on day 21 of the luteal phase of the previous cycle, down-regulation is achieved, and then hMG is given after estradiol suppression is documented. Luteal support with exogenously administered progesterone is important in GnRHa based protocols, as luteal insufficiency is otherwise likely to occur.

Oocyte Retrieval

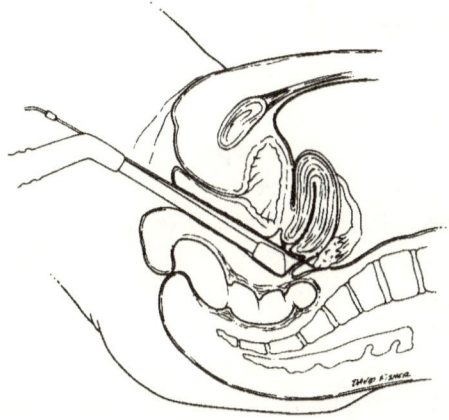

When GnRHa down-regulation is used, oocyte maturation is usually attained at a mean follicle diameter of 18-19 mm. Follicular development is monitored by serum estradiol levels and ultrasound measurements. Oocyte retrieval is performed 34-36 hours following HCG administration. HCG administration results in resumption of oocyte meiotic division and extrusion of the first polar body. Oocyte recovery therefore is scheduled at an interval sufficient to allow oocyte maturation, but before egg release. Transvaginal ultrasound guided oocyte recovery is now the standard procedure for egg retrieval in most IVF centers. This technique is less invasive and increases oocyte yield over other methods used previously.

Intravenous sedation is adequate and appropriate for transvaginal oocyte retrieval. For tubal transfer procedures, some centers will retrieve oocytes transvaginally, and then perform laparoscopy to transfer gametes. Exposure of oocytes to CO_2 is minimized and may improve success rates.

Fertilization

Oocyte Classification

Following oocyte aspiration the eggs are counted, graded and classified using high-quality dissecting or inverted microscopes. Oocyte classification is based on characteristics including the extent of dispersal of the corona radiata and cumulus and the presence or absence of a nuclear membrane or polar body. A mature pre ovulatory oocyte displays extensive dispersal of the surrounding granulosa cells, with an expanded cumulus and corona radiata. Presence of the first polar body indicates that an oocyte is in metaphase II.

Mature pre-ovulatory oocytes usually are pre-incubated for two to eight hours before insemination to allow equilibration in media and to improve fertilization rates. Immature oocytes may benefit from 22-36 hours of *in-vitro* maturation before insemination, and intermediate oocytes may be pre-incubated for 12-24 hours. Recent advances in oocyte culture have improved fertilization rates, especially in male-factor couples. Using a culture system of media droplets under sterile mineral oil stabilizes temperature fluctuations.

Sperm Processing

Fresh ejaculates are allowed to liquefy for 30-60 minutes at room temperature before processing. Sperm are washed twice in culture media and then re-suspended in the same medium. Sperm are incubated for five to seven hours under the same conditions as the eggs, during which time the immotile cells settle out to the bottom leaving an enriched motile fraction of sperm in the supernatant. Sperm are washed at low centrifugation speeds (200 g vs. 600 g) and re-suspended in culture media to concentrate the final yield. Some centers prefer a swim-up technique in which sperm are centrifuged and allowed to swim up into the supernatant layer. Others have popularized the use of Percoll gradients for motile sperm separation.

Insemination of oocytes in IVF

Before insemination, the motility and total number of sperm remaining in suspension are determined. Aliquots of the motile fraction are transferred to the culture dishes containing the eggs. Approximately 100,000 to 500,000 motile sperm are added to each dish containing culture media and eggs (Figure 1). Oligospermic males are treated using a modification of the IVF protocols. Inseminations are carried out with up to 500,000 motile sperm per egg.

Evaluation of Fertilization

After 16-18 hours of incubation, eggs are mechanically stripped of adherent corona radiata cells by passing the eggs through a hand-drawn glass micropipette. Eggs are then classified as fertilized or unfertilized. The success of fertilization is dependent on the concentration and motility of the motile sperm present. Evaluation of eggs shortly after fertilization is critical since certain abnormalities may occur. Fertilization of the egg by two or more sperm results in polyspermy and more than two pronuclei. For obvious reasons, polyspermic eggs are not transferred back to the uterus.

Growth and Development

Fertilized eggs are transferred to a growth medium after evaluation of fertilization. Embryos are evaluated for cleavage and growth rates over the next 24-36 hours. Normally developing embryos have divided to the two-cell stage within 24 hours. Embryos generally are replaced in the uterus at the four-cell to six-cell stage.

Embryo Transfer

IVF-ET approximates the tubal functions of reproduction: oocyte retrieval, incubation of the fertilized oocyte and transport of the embryo to the uterine environment. Yet, despite fertilization rates of 70-80%, and the transfer of pre-embryos that appear to have cleaved normally, the average overall pregnancy rate per embryo transfer remains between 20-30%. This discrepancy between high fertilization rates and relatively low pregnancy rates suggests inefficiency in the process of embryo implantation.

Several factors may play an important role in influencing the success of an embryo transfer: (1) the stage of the embryo at transfer; (2) the synchrony between embryo development and endometrial development; (3) the method and ease of embryo transfer; and (4) the number of embryos transferred.

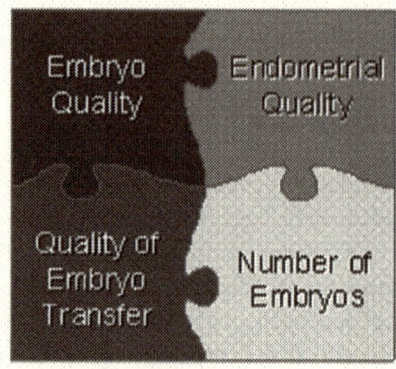

Embryo transfer (ET) generally is done 48 hours after aspiration of oocytes. The cervix is exposed with a speculum, similar to a pap smear exam, and the ecto-cervix gently cleansed with a culture medium. An embryo transfer catheter is loaded in sequence with approximately 10 u L of transfer medium, an air bubble, 10 u L of transfer medium containing all embryos, a second air bubble, and a final 10 u L of transfer medium. The catheter is then introduced into the uterus transcervically, and the embryos are gently transferred. An average of three or four embryos are transferred, depending on the number available, the quality of the embryos, the age, and the wishes of the couple. The catheter is gently with-drawn and returned to the laboratory, where it is carefully examined for retained embryos.

Among those embryos that do implant, there is a 15–30% incidence of mis-carriage. This is similar to the overall spontaneous miscarriage rate that occurs in normally fertile couples and reflects the biological limits of pregnancy exhibited by humans.

FACTORS AFFECTING THE SUCCESS OF IVF-ET

Pregnancy rates decrease between the ages of 35 and 40, and then drop off mark-edly after age 40. Miscarriage rates of IVF-ET pregnancies increase steadily with age, from 18% at ages 25-29, to 29% at age 40. Figure 3 demonstrates the impact of age on fertility:

FIGURE 3
Impact of Female Age on Fertility Outcome

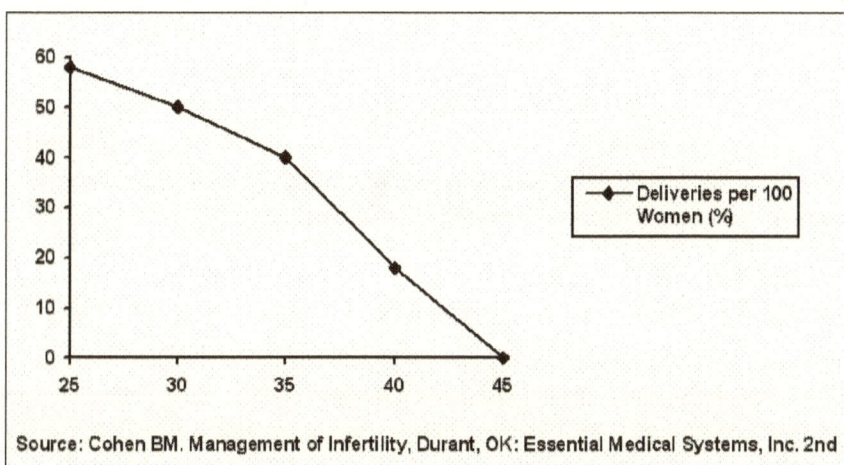

Source: Cohen BM. Management of Infertility, Durant, OK: Essential Medical Systems, Inc. 2nd

The number of embryos transferred may have a dramatic effect on the pregnancy rate. As the number of embryos transferred increases from one to three, the mean pregnancy rate increases from 12 to 24 to 33%. In order to minimize the impact of multiple births and the excessive cost and burden on health care systems dealing with multiple pregnancies, a conservative number of embryos are usually transferred.

The number of IVF cycles that a couple undergoes influences their overall (cumulative) probability of pregnancy. The probability of pregnancy in a second or subsequent cycle does not decline if the first cycle was unsuccessful. While the probability of clinical pregnancy during the first cycle may be 15-30%, the cumulative probability of pregnancy reaches 60-70% after three to six cycles.

Paternal Age

Paternal age is thought to affect fertility and possibly pregnancy loss. There is a striking decline in the conceptions occurring within 6 months according to the age of the husband. Part of this decline in fertility may be due to diminished coital frequency, but any given level of intercourse frequency the proportion of conceptions was higher for husbands under the age of 25 than those 25 and over, with a marked reduction in the proportion of conceptions for those aged 35 and over. Whether this effect of paternal age on fertility is independent of the effect of maternal age, however, has not been determined.

Although the ages of the father and the mother have been found to contribute equally to the risk of late fetal deaths, the evidence for a paternal age effect on the risk of spontaneous miscarriages is conflicting. Some studies have found that advanced paternal age may increase the occurrence of such chromosomal abnormalities as trisomy 21, but others have reported no paternal age effect once adjustments were made for maternal age. The prevalence of certain autosomal dominant disorders, e.g., achondroplasia, has nevertheless been shown to rise with paternal age, even when corrected for maternal age.

GAMETE INTRAFALLOPIAN TRANSFER (GIFT)

Gamete intrafallopian transfer (GIFT) is a method where oocytes and sperm are transferred to one or both fallopian tubes, usually by means of laparoscopically directed tubal cannulation. Thus, fertilization occurs *in-vivo* or naturally in the body. Asch and colleagues reported the first successful pregnancy from GIFT in 1984.

Controlled ovarian stimulation combined with intrauterine insemination (COS-IUI) has often been employed prior to or as an alternative to GIFT. Success rates with COS-IUI, however, vary widely, and most studies demonstrate an improved pregnancy rate with GIFT when compared with COS-IUI. The better pregnancy rates with GIFT are thought to be due to failure of sperm-egg interaction or failure of uniform follicular rupture in COS-IUI. Despite the enhanced efficacy of GIFT in achieving pregnancy, many centers recommend completing two to three cycle of COS-IUI because GIFT is more expensive and requires laparoscopy.

Superovulation may lead to an excessive number of follicles and the risk of ovarian hyperstimulation syndrome. If superovulation develops the treatment may be cancelled and pregnancy avoided to prevent multiple gestation and hyperstimulation syndrome. Superovulation may also be converted to IVF if concerns regarding excessive oocytes exist, allowing for control of the number of embryos transferred.

Indications

The major indications for GIFT include endometriosis unresponsive to therapy, unexplained infertility, and abnormalities of cervical mucus. Women whose partners have oligoasthenospermia (low sperm counts and/or movement) have lower pregnancy rates with GIFT.

Procedures

Patient preparation, ovulation induction and oocyte retrieval (usually by ultrasound guided egg aspiration) are performed in the same fashion as for IVF-ET. General anesthesia is induced and laparoscopy performed wherein gamete transfer is accomplished through a small separate incision site. Approximately 500,000 to 1,000,000 sperm along with oocytes, separated by a bubble in the transfer catheter, are gently discharged in the fallopian tube after the transfer catheter has been placed approximately 3 cm into the tube. In women younger than 35 years of age, only three or four mature oocytes usually are transferred; however, more oocytes may be transferred in women older than 35 without significantly increasing the rate of multiple pregnancies. Interestingly, it does not seem to matter if all gametes are placed in one tube or split between both tubes. Oocytes not transferred may be incubated with sperm *in-vitro* to provide some index of the couple's capability to achieve fertilization, and these embryos may be cryopreserved for later transfer.

Certain apparent advantages of GIFT include *in-vivo* fertilization and less need for the specialized equipment and trained personnel required for IVF. Some have combined GIFT with diagnostic and operative laparoscopy. After laparoscopic aspiration of oocytes, procedures such as lysis of adhesions, ablation of endometriosis and excision of fibroids have been successfully completed before GIFT, and acceptable ongoing pregnancy rates of 24-35% have been reported. Disadvantages of GIFT include the loss of information regarding fertilization (unless IVF with excess oocytes or pregnancy results), the risks of surgery with laparoscopy and the need for general anesthesia. Currently, GIFT has lower success rates than IVF in cases of maternal antisperm antibodies and severe male-factor infertility, and should not be performed when there is significant tubal factor or pelvic adhesions present.

ZYGOTE INTRAFALLOPIAN TRANSFER (ZIFT)

Zygote intrafallopian transfer (ZIFT) is laparoscopic transfer of one or two cell embryos into the fallopian tube after oocyte fertilization *in-vitro*. Indications and patient selection criteria for ZIFT are similar to those for GIFT. Studies have demonstrated that ZIFT is appropriate for couples in which the woman has patency of at least one tube and there is severe male-factor infertility, immunologic infertility, and some cases of unexplained infertility.

The ZIFT protocol involves controlled ovarian stimulation, ultrasonically guided transvaginal oocyte aspiration, *in-vitro* fertilization of oocytes, and then laparoscopic or transcervical tubal embryo transfer. Highlighted in this protocol is the need for two operative procedures: oocyte retrieval followed 1 day later by embryo transfer. Pool employed ZIFT in couples with non tubal infertility and reported an overall clinical pregnancy rate of 40% with a delivery or ongoing pregnancy rate of 34%, compared with concurrent IVF-ET cycles for women with tubal factor having rates of 21% and 15% respectively.

Advantages

Certain advantages of ZIFT over GIFT should be balanced against the requirement for two operative procedures for ZIFT with their medical, financial and logistical drawbacks. ZIFT has advantages for treatment of severe male-factor infertility because it can be established whether each oocyte is fertilized. The replacement of known embryos has resulted in improved pregnancy rates for this indication. In couples with severe oligoasthenospermia and poor *in-vitro* fertilization, ZIFT with embryos obtained from oocyte micromanipulation have resulted in pregnancies.

EMBRYO CRYOPRESERVATION

The efficiency of modern superovulation regimens for IVF-GIFT has provided multiple embryos for transfer. The transfer of multiple embryos has increased the clinical pregnancy rate; however the use of larger numbers of embryos (greater than two) also raises risks for multiple pregnancy. Advances in cryobiology have demonstrated promise for lowering the cost and risk of IVF-GIFT procedures by decreasing the number of egg recovery cycles per pregnancy while limiting multiple pregnancies.

The goal of an enhanced cumulative pregnancy rate per oocyte retrieval has been realized with cryopreservation. The general principles and methods of freezing embryos involve multiple steps and are different depending upon the stage of embryo development. Generally, embryos are initially exposed to a permeating cryoprotectant agent such as 1,2-propanediol for one-cell to four-cell embryos, or glycerol for blastocysts. Seeding is used to induce ice crystal formation and to prevent excessive cooling before reaching the storage temperature of liquid nitrogen (-196° C). Subsequently, embryos may be thawed to room temperature, and the permeating cryoprotectant removed before transfer of embryos to a physiological environment for the resumption of development.

Initial reports of success in transferring thawed embryos were somewhat discouraging with low pregnancy rates. Recently, the problems with freezing and thawing have improved and successful pregnancy rates have improved. Additionally, new insights into uterine and endometrial preparation have also led to better outcomes. Some programs now report almost identical success in transferring fresh or frozen/thawed embryos.

INTRACYTOPLASMIC SPERM INJECTION (ICSI)

Although conventional IVF has proven useful in the treatment of significant male-factor infertility, severe sperm abnormalities still may result in fertilization failure. Recently, microsurgical techniques have been developed for these difficult cases, and have proven successful even for individuals with sperm concentrations lower than 1 million per mL. Oocyte micromanipulation is an attempt to affect fertilization by enabling sperm to traverse the barrier posed by the zona pellucida.

The first, and probably least, traumatic technique involves creation of a gap in the zona pellucida, thus facilitating the entrance of motile sperm into the perivitelline space. Variations of this procedure have been described ranging from chemical "drilling" with acidic Tyrode's solution, to mechanical incision of the zona.

The most recent and most successful approach entails the direct microinjection of a single sperm into the ooplasm: intracytoplasmic sperm injection (ICSI). This procedure involves the insertion of a single spermatozoon, regardless of its motility and/or acrosomal status. This direct injection technique established pregnancies in 1992, and continues to hold promise for the treatment of sperm defects of recognition, binding, fusion, and penetration of the oolema.

ASSISTED HATCHING

Another novel application of zona micromanipulation is "assisted hatching," a technique applied to normal embryos before transfer. Based on the observation that cleaved embryos with thinned areas on their zona have higher implantation rates, Cohen hypothesized that one factor limiting success rates in IVF may be a failure of blastocyst hatching from the zona, a prerequisite for implantation. A prospective, randomized study was performed, comparing assisted hatching with transfer of zona-intact embryos. The implantation rate for the assisted hatching group was 22%, compared with 13% per embryo for the control group (P<.05). Further investigation is ongoing and may lead to an overall improvement of success rates following IVF.

EGG DONATION

The desire of an increasing population of women to have children in their late 30's and 40's has prompted options to increase the success of achieving this goal. Egg quality in women decreases as a function of age and the efficiency of reproductive success decreases in the same order with an increase of miscarriage due to genetic errors. Egg donation started in the late 1980's as an alternative to supply women capable of carrying a pregnancy with a supply of young, healthy eggs that maintain their high level of reproductive efficiency. Success rates for pregnancy are known to increase dramatically with the use of this treatment option.

PREIMPLANTATION GENETIC TESTING (PGD)

Microsurgical manipulations of gametes and embryos may also be used as diagnostic and possibly therapeutic procedures as well. Biopsies of the polar body or embryonic blastomere can be performed before implantation in women at high risk for genetic disease and be coupled with advanced genetic techniques to identify oocytes or embryos that carry specific genetic markers. Any unaffected embryos can then be transferred.

GESTATIONAL SURROGACY

Another advance in reproductive technology is the use of gestational surrogacy in IVF-ET. These are among the most fascinating as well as legally and ethically complicated components of current reproductive technology. They are also the most exciting because of the overall high success rates achieved.

Using in-vitro fertilization (IVF), the union of the couple's sperm and oocyte results in an embryo transferred to the woman's uterus with the genetic complement of the infant being that of the couple who intend on being parents. There are two basic variations which include: (1) transferring the genetic embryo of the intended parents into a gestational surrogate; and (2) donor eggs used for women with primary or secondary gonadal failure (e.g. peri-menopause, premature ovarian failure, gonadal dysgenesis), or for those with repeated assisted conception failures or those with inheritable genetic traits.

Women in this circumstance usually have an indication for a gestational "host" that includes hysterectomy, incompetent cervix, scarring within the uterine cavity (asherman's syndrome), an abnormal uterine configuration that is not surgically correctable (i.e. unicornualte uterus, T-shaped uterus, etc.) or uterine disease such as Adenomyosis.

EMBRYO DONATION

After years of successful in-vitro fertilization procedures have been performed, couples may find themselves with "extra" embryos. Embryos are the property of the couples and they may have their embryos destroyed or donate these embryos to other couples desiring children, but unable to do so. This has opened up a new reproductive option for couples called embryo donation.

Candidates for embryo adoption include virtually anyone willing to accept a child who has no genetic ties. These might be couples who were otherwise willing to adopt a child but were unable to do so for finanacial or social reasons. Some other examples of candidates for embryo donation include women with poor egg/embryo quality; adoptive couples who wish they could experience pregnancy and breast feeding their child; couples who have genetic family traits that they wish to avoid and therefore welcome the traits of quality embryos.

Use of donor embryos tends to be significantly less expensive than IVF since the expensive components of care (follicle stimulation, egg retrieval and fertilization) have been completed. Overall success is high since donor embryo quality tends to be better than average. Their sibling embryos created the successful pregnancies that fulfilled the family dream for the couple that generated the embryos.

SUMMARY

The role of assisted reproductive technology has given hope to many couples in their quest for parenthood where options for success were minimal or nonexistent. This will continue to be a dynamic specialty of ever-changing technology to enable and increase this opportunity for couples around the world to enjoy the privileges of parenthood.

Conclusion

MAGNITUDE OF THE PROBLEM

By using the clinical definition of infertility, national surveys estimate that 15 percent of U.S. couples have difficulty conceiving a pregnancy. An additional 15-40 percent of recognized pregnancies end in spontaneous miscarriage. Pregnancy loss may also occur before a woman is aware that she is pregnant. It is estimated that as many as 60 percent of fertilized eggs may not survive implantation.

As couples have delayed childbearing to later years, medical conditions create a higher rate of reproductive failure. The conception that was achieved spontaneously may later associate with miscarriage, then blur into infertility.

THERAPEUTIC OPPORTUNITIES

It is important to emphasize that reproductive failure can be a multifactorial disorder involving both female and male factors. Many of these causative factors may be acting independently and all couples warrant a thorough evaluation.

Random genetic or developmental abnormalities of the embryo may be responsible for a substantial proportion of pregnancy losses. Advanced maternal age, maternal infections and medical illness are among the few important causes of spontaneous miscarriages. Environmental factors may also be associated with genetically normal and abnormal miscarriages. Hormone support and anticoagulant therapy for autoimmune and blood clotting disorders provide benefit. Anatomic reasons for miscarriage offer the possibility of surgical correction and dramatic success.

The world of assisted reproductive technology offers many optimistic opportunities to both diagnose and achieve an ongoing pregnancy. Egg donation, pre-implantation genetic testing of embryos and gestational surrogacy offer significant hope for couples with reproductive loss.

PLANNING FOR THE FUTURE

A physician evaluation is essential for patients with pregnancy loss. A thorough clinical investigation should be pursued in an effort to uncover all of the known causes of recurrent pregnancy loss.

Couples should be reassured to know that effective therapy associates with a successful pregnancy outcome in over 60% of couples. Relieving stress, fear, and frustration can improve a couple's relationship and their reproductive outcome.

Ongoing investigational efforts in miscarriage will lead to the development of more effective treatments for successful outcomes.

Index

978-0-595-35715-ⁿ
0-595-35715-6